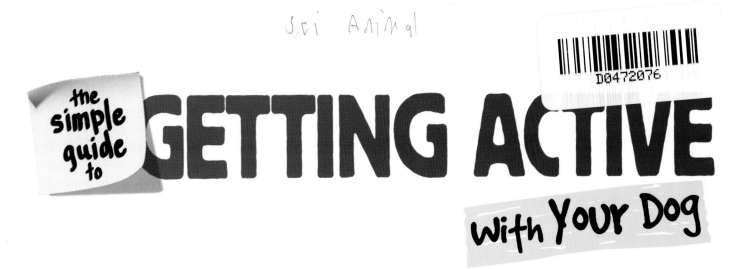

the simple guide to GETTING ACTIVE
with Your Dog

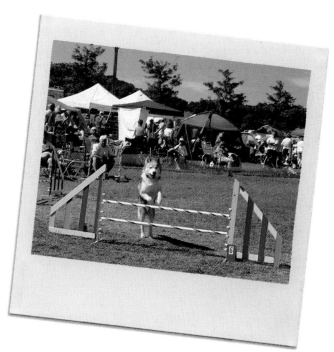

t.f.h.

T.F.H. Publications, Inc.

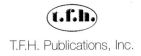

Margaret H. Bonham

Distributed in the UNITED STATES to the Pet Trade by T.F.H. Publications, Inc., 1 TFH Plaza, Neptune City, NJ 07753; on the Internet at www.tfh.com; in CANADA by Rolf C. Hagen Inc., 3225 Sartelon St., Montreal, Quebec H4R 1E8; Pet Trade by H & L Pet Supplies Inc., 27 Kingston Crescent, Kitchener, Ontario N2B 2T6; in ENGLAND by T.F.H. Publications, PO Box 74, Havant PO9 5TT; in AUSTRALIA AND THE SOUTH PACIFIC by T.F.H. (Australia), Pty. Ltd., Box 149, Brookvale 2100 N.S.W., Australia; in NEW ZEALAND by Brooklands Aquarium Ltd., 5 McGiven Drive, New Plymouth, RD1 New Zealand; in SOUTH AFRICA by Rolf C. Hagen S.A. (PTY.) LTD., P.O. Box 201199, Durban North 4016, South Africa; in Japan by T.F.H. Publications. Published by T.F.H. Publications, Inc.

Manufactured in the United States of America by T.F.H. Publications, Inc.

Contents

Assessing Your Dog's Health Page 17-22

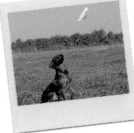

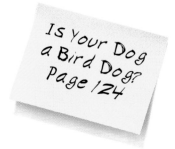
Is Your Dog
a Bird Dog?
Page 124

On the
Road
Page 159

Part One
Getting Started

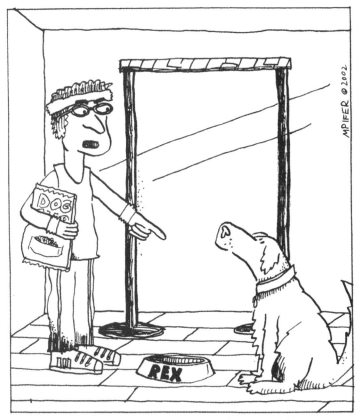

"I don't care if you have opposable thumbs or not! You're going to do fifteen chin ups or no dinner!"

Choosing the Right Activity for You and Your Dog

One hundred and twenty-five thousand years ago, the relationship between humans and wolves began to evolve. Domestication produced a modified wolf that we now call the dog. There is little doubt that ancient peoples discovered the dog's usefulness in hunting and protection. Humans, encouraged by the dog's willingness to be a helper, bred the dog for desirable traits. Dogs herded and protected stock, carried loads, ridded farms and cities of vermin, and even aided in transportation.

Sadly, within the last hundred years, the dog has become largely unemployed. Dogs were bred for a purpose—a hundred years or even a thousand years will not change that instinct. If you thumb through

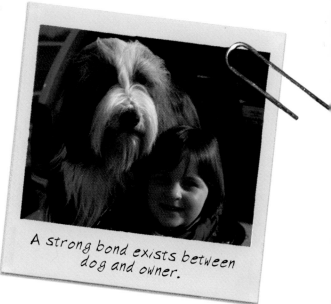

A strong bond exists between dog and owner.

the American Kennel Club's *The Complete Dog Book*, you will find that the dog breeds are separated into distinct groups or categories. Other kennel clubs around the world have somewhat different groupings, but the categories are there. In *The Complete Dog Book*, you will find groups such as Hounds, Working, Sporting, Terriers, etc.–a testimony to the type of work for which the dog was originally bred. Even mixed breeds carry some traits of their working ancestors–how could they not?

Consequently, some dogs are throwbacks to a time when they were useful. This frustration often expresses itself in a dog's undesirable behavior. Every year, 5 million unwanted pets are euthanized at animal shelters, many because of behavioral issues. This is not a reflection on the dog as much as the owner. These owners expect the dog to be a self-maintenance pet.

Dogs, like humans, are not content to be idle and need a purpose in their lives. This book offers ways to fill this void. It gives you practical ways for training your dog, a synopsis of each of the sports, and more information on how to get involved further.

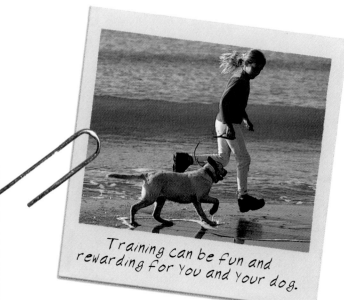

Training can be fun and rewarding for you and your dog.

Benefits of Dog Sports

Why bother training your dog at all? There are several good reasons to train a dog, not the least of which is control. At best, an untrained dog is an obnoxious nuisance. At worst, an untrained dog can be dangerous. Everyone knows the dangers posed by large, aggressive dogs, but even small dog bites can be serious. Even when dogs are not aggressive, they can still be dangerous. Large, boisterous dogs can knock down children and seniors, and they are a handful to walk or take in the car.

Training can be fun and rewarding for both you and your dog. When you are participating in a sport or activity with your dog, you are training him, whether you realize it or not. Sports quickly become fun, rather than just training. Most organized dog sports require a small amount of obedience, but do not require the rigors or precision of competitive obedience–although that is certainly open to you, if you wish.

Training for any activity helps strengthen the human-dog bond. Not surprisingly, most owners who participate in canine sports report a closer relationship with their dogs. This isn't surprising, because the owner actually is spending more time with the dog. The positive interaction helps the dog bond more closely to his owner.

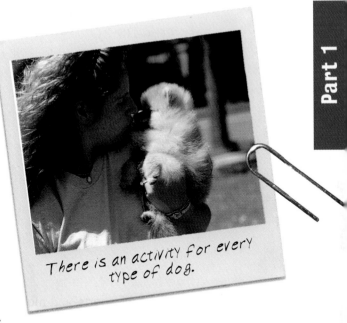

There is an activity for every type of dog.

Any type of training activity also helps release excess energy. A tired dog is a happy dog, and one less likely to cause mischief. The dog focuses energy on the exercise at hand and becomes more settled and tractable. Because dog sports combine training and exercise, the dog learns to listen to your commands even when not performing. Most dog owners remark on how their dogs "settle down" when given a job to do. Training in any dog sport also often helps with problems due to boredom and lack of self-confidence. Owners of problem dogs typically report that their dogs become better behaved. Nervous and shy dogs become more confident. Owners who have reported their dog's destructive behavior often see the behavior lessen or become eliminated entirely.

No, it doesn't happen overnight. The progress is gradual as the negative behavior starts to diminish. Not all negative behaviors can be controlled with activities but many can. Dog owners who want to enjoy positive relationships with their dogs will have nothing to lose by getting involved in sports and outdoor activities.

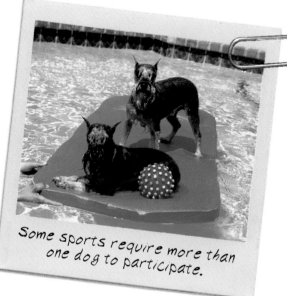

Some sports require more than one dog to participate.

One or More Dogs?

You need not have several dogs to participate in most dog sports. In fact, most activities are intended for one-on-one training, although a few, such as sledding, require a number of dogs. Dogs do not need to be a particular breed either; they just need to be in good health and have a willing owner.

If you have several dogs, pick just one to try the new activity. Don't try training the other dogs until you have confidently trained the first one. An exception to this is if more than one person in your family wishes to try the same sport. Then, by all means, have the other person choose a dog to train and the two of you can train together. Training dogs can be a fun family event.

How Many Dogs?

The following is a table of the number of dogs required for each sport or activity.

Sport or Activity	One or More	Two or More
Obedience	X	
Agility	X	
Tracking	X	
Field Trials		X
Hunting Tests	X	
Herding	X	
Earthdog	X	
Lure Coursing	X	
Carting	X	
Skijoring	X	
Weightpulling	X	
Sledding		X
Backpacking	X	
Flyball	X	
Flying Disc	X	
Freestyle Dancing	X	
Schutzhund	X	

Mixed Breed or Purebred?

Many of the sports mentioned here allow both mixed breed and purebreds to participate. Some activities are breed specific, such as lure coursing or earthdog trials. These activities are recognized through national governing bodies such as the American Kennel Club (AKC) and the specific breed clubs that sponsor their titles.

Mixed Breed or Purebred?

The following is a list of activities and the restrictions on participation. An asterisk (*) means that AKC limits participation to purebred dogs only, but there are other options for competition.

Sport or Activity	Breed Restrictions, If Any:
Obedience	None*
Agility	None*
Tracking	None*
Field Trials	Beagles, Basset Hounds, Dachshunds, all pointers, all retrievers, most spaniels
Hunting Tests	Pointers, flushing spaniels, retrievers, standard Poodles
Herding	Herding Group breeds, Rottweilers, Samoyed
Earth Dog	Small terriers, Dachshunds
Lure Coursing	Afghan Hounds, Basenji, Borzoi, Greyhounds, Ibizan Hounds, Irish Wolfhounds, Norwegian Elkhounds, Pharaoh Hounds, Rhodesian Ridgebacks, Salukis, Scottish Deerhounds, Whippets
Carting	None
Skijoring	None
Weightpulling	None
Sledding	None
Backpacking	None
Flyball	None
Flying Disc	None
Freestyle	None
Schutzhund	None

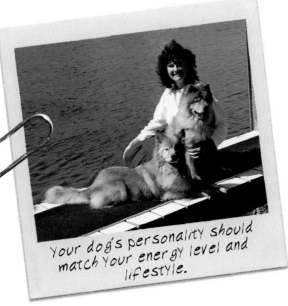

Your dog's personality should match your energy level and lifestyle.

Your Lifestyle and Activity Level

Obviously, some activities depend on your lifestyle and activity level. Some activities, such as sledding and herding, require special equipment and conditions. Your neighbors (to say nothing of the law) may object to the sheep pen in the back of your suburban residence! However, some activities require minimal equipment; flying disc requires a few flying discs; freestyle dancing requires a portable stereo and music.

Where you live, your level of commitment, and activity level will factor into what sports are right for you and your dog. You'll be more motivated to stay with the activity if it is something you can do easily, as opposed to one that takes hours of preparation and travel. Many training facilities offer obedience, tracking, and agility training, and there are many clubs that host obedience and agility trials.

How much work is required? Again, it depends on your level of commitment. All dog sports, short of playing fetch, require some commitment in order to become competitive. Select a few from the list that interest you and try them. You'll get a quick understanding of what type of commitment is required.

How Much Does It Cost?

The cost of a particular activity depends on the equipment required, the number of dogs, and the level of commitment. Some activities, such as agility, can become very time-intensive and costly, depending on the number of trials entered. Sledding, for example, is very expensive and equipment intensive. Note that any activity can quickly become expensive if you decide to travel or become seriously competitive.

Competition or Just for Fun?

Most of the sports mentioned have competitive events. Many dog owners intend to try these sports out just for fun, but not surprisingly, become hooked and quickly begin to think about competition.

Cost

The following table ranks the activities in terms of cost to get started. Any activity, if pursued with competition in mind, can become expensive quickly.

$—inexpensive $$$—expensive

$$—moderately expensive $$$$—costly

Sport and Activity Cost

Obedience $—$$$	Skijoring $—$$$
Agility $—$$$	(Less if you own ski equipment)
Tracking $—$$$	Weightpulling $—$$
Field Trials $$—$$$	Sledding $$$—$$$$
Hunting Tests $$—$$$	Backpacking $—$$
Herding $$—$$$$	(Less if you own backpacking equipment)
Earth Dog $$—$$$	Flyball $—$$$
Lure Coursing $—$$	Flying Disc $—$$
Carting $$	Freestyle $—$$
	Schutzhund $$—$$$

If you decide to do the activity just for fun, that's okay. You and your dog will have the time of your lives. Nevertheless, you will always have the option of competing if you're ever interested.

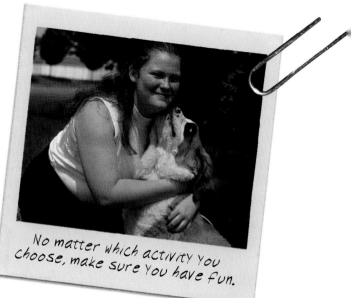

No matter which activity you choose, make sure you have fun.

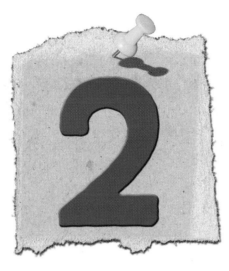

Canine Couch Potatoes— Do You Have One?

Many of the activities discussed in this book require that your dog be at a certain level of physical condition *before* starting the activity. The average housepet is usually overweight and not in condition. Before you begin any activity or exercise regimen with your dog, talk to your veterinarian. Your vet may suggest ways of trimming down your dog and certain exercises. He may wish to x-ray your dog's hips and elbows to see if your dog is sound enough for the activity, especially if it is strenuous.

Your Dog's Condition

If you would like to start a physical activity or sport with your dog, he should not be overweight. Overweight dogs are slow and prone to injury. As in

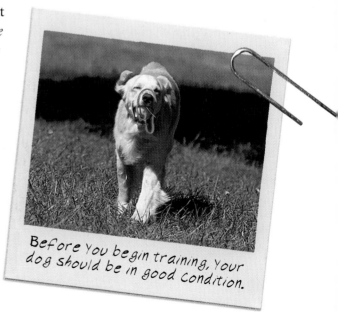

Before you begin training, your dog should be in good condition.

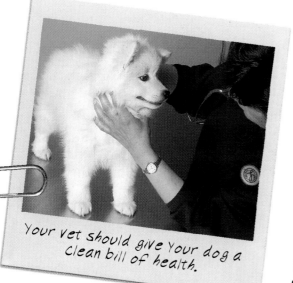

Your vet should give your dog a clean bill of health.

humans, obesity in dogs is unhealthy. An overweight dog is at a much higher risk of developing weight-associated diseases. Jumping, pulling, and other activities are more difficult and cause more stress on joints when a dog is overweight.

Although weighing your dog may provide a good guideline when comparing him to the breed standard, it does not provide a good measure of a dog's fitness. Body structure varies from dog to dog, even within a breed, so weight should only be used as one indicator.

The best way to determine your dog's fitness is to put your thumbs on his spine and feel the ribs with your outstretched fingers. You should be able to feel your dog's spine, ribs, and ribcage easily. Moving your hands toward the tail, you should also be able to feel the pelvis. If you

Getting Your Dog in Shape

Before beginning any conditioning program, it's always a good idea to consult your veterinarian. Your vet may be able to suggest exercises and a diet to keep your dog in good shape.

Here's how to begin exercising:

• Start slowly and gradually build up. Don't overstress your dog. Start with a mile or less and don't go full speed. Slowly build up the mileage.

• Go slowly on concrete and asphalt. These surfaces can injure joints. Try to avoid these surfaces, if possible; however, if you ride, walk, or jog on concrete or asphalt, consider using booties to protect your dog's sensitive pads. You can obtain cordura booties from an outfitter that sells dog backpacks or mushing equipment.

• Be extra careful in warm temperatures. If your dog is panting or having trouble keeping up, slow down or rest.

• Give your dog enough water to prevent dehydration.

• Don't exercise when it is too hot. This depends on your dog's ability to tolerate temperature and humidity. Humidity intensifies high temperatures. Generally, any temperature over 75°F is too warm for exercise. Activities such as sledding usually require temperatures below 60°F.

• Know the signs of heat exhaustion, heat stroke, and dehydration. Never push your dog to the point of exhaustion.

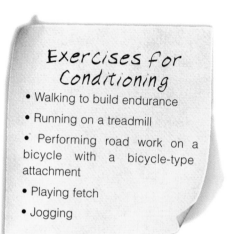

Exercises for Conditioning

- Walking to build endurance
- Running on a treadmill
- Performing road work on a bicycle with a bicycle-type attachment
- Playing fetch
- Jogging

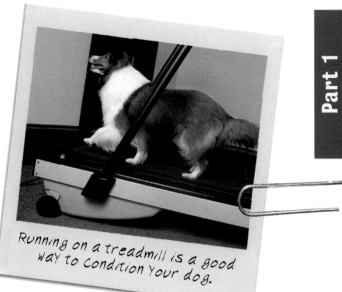

Running on a treadmill is a good way to condition your dog.

cannot feel the spine, ribs, or pelvis, or must search to feel them (that is, if they are heavily padded), your dog is probably too fat. Consult your veterinarian, who may recommend a special low-calorie diet.

The Right Nutrition

Your dog's diet depends largely on age, activity level, and condition. Just as a human athlete doesn't eat junk food, don't feed your dog the canine equivalent of potato chips. High-performance dogs require high-performance diets.

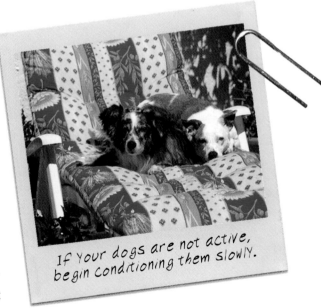

If your dogs are not active, begin conditioning them slowly.

The food you choose should have a statement that says "complete and nutritionally balanced" or that the food meets the guidelines as set forth by the Association of American Feed Control Officials (AAFCO). The AAFCO has established guidelines for dogs' and puppies' nutritional needs. Most major dog food companies comply with AAFCO regulations, but you should check regardless of the brand or manufacturer.

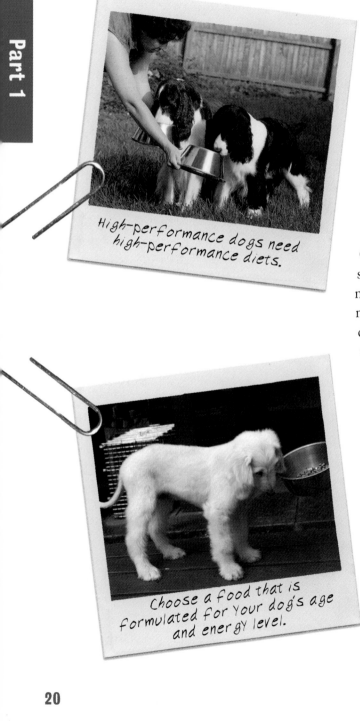

High-performance dogs need high-performance diets.

Choose a food that is formulated for your dog's age and energy level.

Protein, Fat, and Carbohydrates

The first two ingredients in any dog food should include the protein source: chicken, beef, poultry-by-products, lamb meal, etc. Don't shy away from foods with by-products; they are excellent sources of protein and should not be overlooked. You should also consider chicken meal or poultry by-product meal, as they are simply the same ingredients with the water removed.

The quality of the dog food ingredients depends solely on the manufacturer. The definition of "by-products," for example, leaves much open to interpretation. Chicken by-products from one source may be far superior in quality to chicken by-products from another manufacturer. Some by-products have better quality nutrition than their actual meat source. The AAFCO definition of meat can include heart and tongue, not just the muscle meat. Also, the AAFCO definition of "poultry" is broad. Don't be fooled into thinking that because you bought a dog food that says "poultry," that it doesn't include livers or gizzards.

Protein is a very important nutrient for dogs. Besides providing 4 Kcals (kilocalories or "calories") of energy per gram, it provides the building blocks necessary for the formation of muscle, connective tissue, coat, nails, skin, blood, and internal organs. Protein is very important for growing puppies, active adults, and pregnant females. Older dogs require protein, too. Don't limit protein unless your older dog is obese or has kidney problems. Your veterinarian can recommend an appropriate diet in these circumstances.

Protein can come from a variety of animals and plants. Animal protein is more complete than plant protein, meaning that it contains the correct balance of amino acids for a dog to live on. Plant protein usually comes from a variety of sources, if you choose a diet that is strictly vegetarian.

The AAFCO's minimum protein requirements for dry dog food are 22 percent for puppy formulas and 18 percent for adult preparations. Note that these are the bare minimum percentages—when you buy a premium dog food, you are more likely to see protein levels somewhere around 25-26 percent for active adult dogs and 27-31 percent for puppies.

Fat is a wonderful energy-dense nutrient at 9 Kcals per gram. Extensive research shows that canine athletes metabolize fat in a way similar to the way human athletes use carbohydrates. Dogs generally do not suffer from high cholesterol, so using animal fat is not a concern. Fat is also important in maintaining a healthy skin and coat. Fat provides insulation from cold and protects organs. It also carries fat-soluble vitamins such as A, D, E, and K.

High-quality fat sources include animal fat. Dogs use fats that are commonly referred to as Omega-6, long-chained fatty acids. They are usually a mixture of saturated (solid) and unsaturated (liquid) fats. Unsaturated fat tends to turn rancid quicker. Typical fat sources include beef, poultry, and "animal fat," which may be a mixture of pork, beef, lamb, and horse fat.

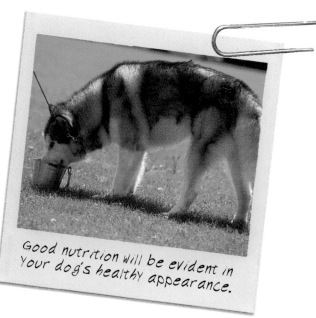

Good nutrition will be evident in your dog's healthy appearance.

The latest nutrition rage has been the Omega-3 fatty acids, touted for their overall health benefits. Common sources include a variety of fish oils and linseed oil. Omega-3 fatty acids are noted to help decrease the risk of developing certain kinds of tumors and cancers and have anti-inflammatory properties. However, you can have too much of a good thing. Tests have shown that too much Omega-3 fatty acids can inhibit blood clotting in humans, and the potential for hemorrhaging with injury may be too great. No more than 4-5 percent of the dry matter weight should be Omega-3 fatty acids. This does not mean you should change your current pet food if it contains Omega-3 fatty acids; rather, you should be careful if you use supplements or if the Omega-3 fatty acids are the primary fat source in the food.

The AAFCO's minimum requirement for fat is 5 percent for adults and 8 percent for puppies. Most dog foods have more because it is an excellent energy source and makes the food more palatable.

The most common carbohydrate sources in pet foods include corn and corn products, rice, and wheat. As a dog becomes more active, fewer carbohydrates and more protein and fat are required. Some dogs have wheat or corn allergies, making barley, rice, or oatmeal an acceptable substitute.

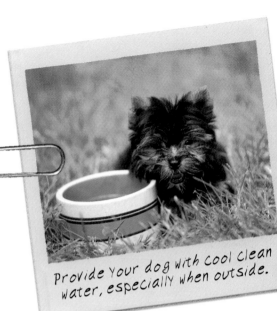

Provide your dog with cool clean water, especially when outside.

Water

Water is the most important nutrient for your dog. No dog can live long without it. Every major system throughout the body uses water. Your dog cannot perform optimally when he is dehydrated. Even mild dehydration can severely affect performance.

Dehydration can occur at any time of the year. During the hot summer months, a dog will drink water to help avoid dehydration, but it can also occur during the winter months, especially if the air is cold and dry. Some dogs may not drink enough water and may have to be coaxed into drinking. You can coax him to drink by flavoring the water with bits of dog food, meat scraps, or beef broth.

Always provide water from a known good source. Streams and creeks may contain giardia or other organisms that may cause severe diarrhea and vomiting.

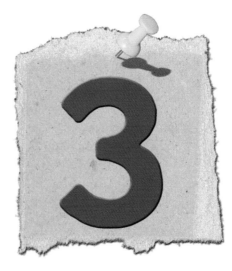

Before You Start

Before you start participating in activities with your dog, make sure she is well trained and receptive to new training. Positive reinforcement is currently a popular training method. Unlike older negative reinforcement methods that relied on avoidance techniques, positive methods rely on praise and food (or some other motivational item).

The most common positive reinforcement techniques use food and praise because most dogs are well motivated by them. However, some dogs are not food motivated; in this case, find a favorite toy or item and use that in training.

Negative reinforcement relies on doing something

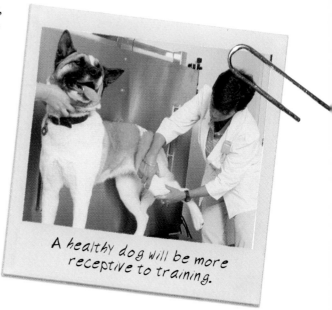

A healthy dog will be more receptive to training.

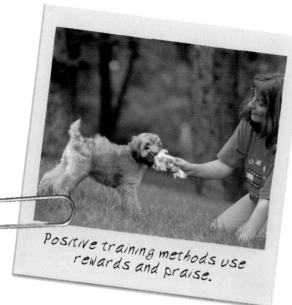

Positive training methods use rewards and praise.

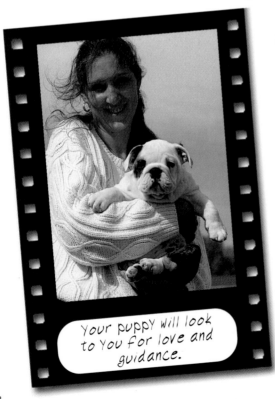

Your puppy will look to you for love and guidance.

that the dog will avoid in order to obtain the correct behavior. Jerking the collar harshly, throwing a shaker can, squirting water, and shouting are all forms of negative reinforcement. Negative reinforcement produces avoidance behavior; that is, the dog wants to avoid the punishment and therefore performs the correct behavior.

Why Positive Methods Work

The problem with using negative reinforcement is that you are using avoidance to shape a behavior. Dogs–and people–perform best when they are motivated to perform. Think of the last time you were made to do something you did not like. If you weren't internally motivated to do a good job, chances are you completed the task adequately at best. Now, think of a task that you enjoyed, one for which you received some kind of reward. The job might have been fun, and you were probably putting forth your best effort.

We all like being rewarded for a job well done–why shouldn't dogs? Positive reinforcement relies on that concept. Because this is a learning experience, your dog will try a number of different actions until she gives you the correct behavior, the one you are looking for. Once she knows the behavior you want–the one that will get the treat, toy, or praise–you'll find her trying to perfect that behavior.

What is a Correction?

This book will be using the words "correct" and "correction" often throughout the text. The definition of correction for our purposes is "anything that causes a dog to cease his current actions in a meaningful manner." It does not mean hit, kick, or yell at your dog. It does not mean jerk and drag the dog around. Correction must be meaningful to your dog in some way; that is, she must associate her current behavior with the action *you've* taken. The correction must also be effective otherwise it is completely meaningless. What you are trying to do is guide your dog into the appropriate responses for a certain set of conditions.

When a dog does something wrong, she often does not understand or has misinterpreted what you have asked her to do. To punish a dog for something she does not understand is misguided. Never punish a dog for a mistake. The dog needs to be corrected and shown the appropriate behavior. For example, your dog jumps up on you every time you enter the house. To stop this behavior, put your dog in a sit/stay and reward her with a treat. Then pet your dog as she sits, shaping the proper greeting behavior. By diverting your dog's bad habits into something positive, you have issued a correction and offered an alternative.

Make Training Fun

We're all motivated to do better when we have fun, so why should dogs be any different? Make the new activity fun, not work, for your dog. Your dog will enjoy the training sessions more if you can make them an upbeat and fun game. Provide a reward or incentive. Toys that give "jackpots," such as treats that are buried inside, work well. Some dogs enjoy playing with tennis balls, flying discs, or other toys. Avoid repetition. Dogs, like people, become tired of the same thing. Vary your training with new commands or tasks and break up sessions with play. Both you and your dog will enjoy this time together.

End your training session on a positive note. If your training session is going poorly, try something the dog

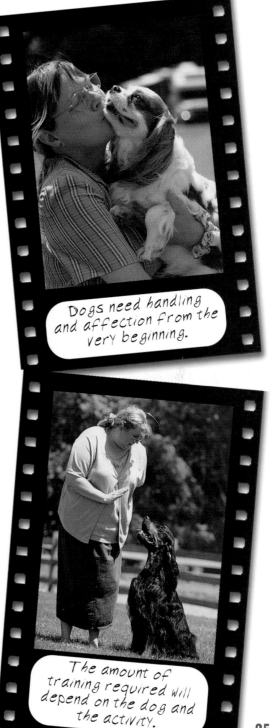

Dogs need handling and affection from the very beginning.

The amount of training required will depend on the dog and the activity.

Part 1

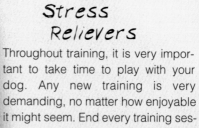

Stress Relievers

Throughout training, it is very important to take time to play with your dog. Any new training is very demanding, no matter how enjoyable it might seem. End every training session positively with a game your dog enjoys. Your dog will look forward to training sessions more often if they are positive and fun.

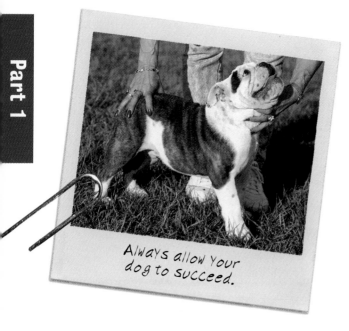

Always allow your dog to succeed.

Reward good behavior with safe treats.

already knows and does well. Once she accomplishes that, end the session. Never end on a sour note.

How Often to Train

The amount of training depends largely on the activity and the dog. Some breeds (and individual dogs) require training every day. Some activities–such as sledding–require conditioning every day or several times a week.

When you first start the activity, you may need to train every day for the first few weeks. If you practice every day, be certain to keep the training sessions short, 5 to 10 minutes, to avoid burnout. If you practice once or twice a week, the sessions should be a bit longer. If the activity requires conditioning, such as sledding or skijoring, start with short distances and slowly work up to longer distances.

Positive Training Techniques

• Never get angry at your dog. This sport thing was *your* idea, not the dog's. If you feel yourself becoming angry or frustrated at your dog—stop. Take a time out. Stop training. Play with your dog, take a walk, or read a book. Don't take your frustration out on your canine partner.

• Become a person your dog will respect. Don't yell and scream when she does something wrong. Don't wheedle and cajole her to get a response to a command. Corrections and praise should be swift and meaningful. Always place yourself above your dog.

• Always reward your dog for coming to you. Never use punishment when your dog returns after running away, or you will be punishing the dog for coming back.

• Never force a frightened dog to do something. The dog may react aggressively and will be more difficult to control in the future.

• Before you can teach a command, you must first have your dog's attention. Always precede the command with your dog's name, such as, "Trixie, come!" not, "Come, Trixie!" Trixie probably did not hear the command before you got her attention.

• Say the command once. Don't yell—your dog is not deaf. Truly deaf dogs should be taught with hand signals instead. Don't repeat the command. You'll be teaching your dog that it is not necessary to obey the first command. Exception to this rule: Teaching the command the first time. Sometimes when teaching the come command, a dog may need some extra positive encouragement. Once the dog learns the command, you don't have to repeat it unless there is a long time between giving the command and the time the action needs to be performed.

• Choose one command and stick with it. Don't say, "Trixie, Jump!" on one jump and then, "Trixie, over!" on another jump.

• Choose one-word commands that don't sound like each other. "Sit down" and "Lie down" are perfect examples of what will confuse your dog. Use the commands "Sit" for "Sit down" and "Down" for "Lie down" instead.

• Don't use the down command in place of "Off." The down command should mean lie down. "Off" should mean all four paws are on the ground.

• Never give a command that you cannot enforce. It's not funny hearing someone say, "Trixie, come! Trixie, come! Trixie get over here! Okay, Trixie, don't come." This shows an obvious lack of control. Always enforce a command. If your dog is not reliable off leash, keep her on a long line until she becomes reliable. For example, if your dog doesn't sit after you give her that command, make her sit.

• Always reward good behavior.

• Always set your dog up for success and never allow her to make a mistake. This is easier than it sounds. Think about what you are teaching your dog, what possible responses she can have, and then be prepared for them. *Remember: It is easier to teach good habits than it is to correct bad ones.*

• Always end a training session on a positive note.

• Take time to play. Your dog needs play time with you to release stress and excess energy.

• Have fun. If neither of you have fun, why bother?

Part Two
Activities for Every Dog

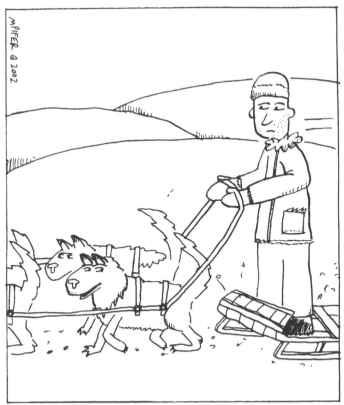

"Ok, five more minutes of this, and then it's our turn on the sled."

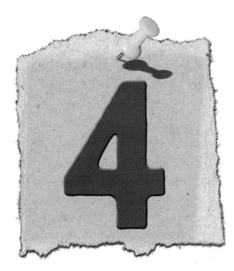

Backpacking

Backpacking in the wilderness is more enjoyable when you take your best friend along. Most dogs enjoy having something to do and carrying their water and treats often adds to the dog's usefulness as well as enjoyment. Indeed, miles of trails await you and your best friend.

Any dog in good condition can backpack. Visit your veterinarian to make sure that your dog is healthy, and free from injuries, joint problems, and bone malformations before beginning. Even healthy older dogs may backpack, provided that you take their age and condition into consideration when exercising. If you have a puppy or a young dog, wait until he is at least 18 months old. Backpacking

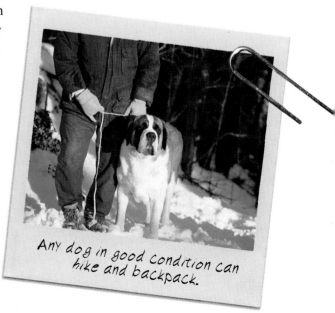

Any dog in good condition can hike and backpack.

Part 2

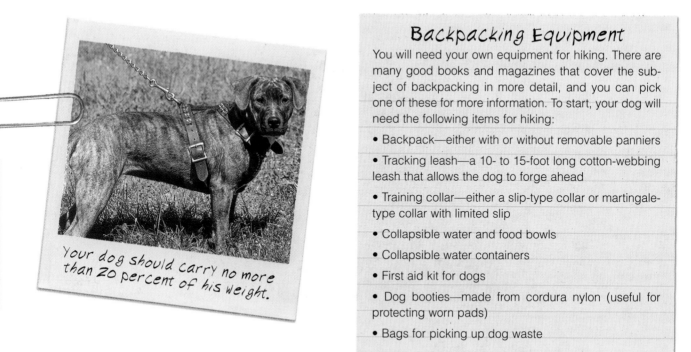

Your dog should carry no more than 20 percent of his weight.

Backpacking Equipment

You will need your own equipment for hiking. There are many good books and magazines that cover the subject of backpacking in more detail, and you can pick one of these for more information. To start, your dog will need the following items for hiking:

• Backpack—either with or without removable panniers

• Tracking leash—a 10- to 15-foot long cotton-webbing leash that allows the dog to forge ahead

• Training collar—either a slip-type collar or martingale-type collar with limited slip

• Collapsible water and food bowls

• Collapsible water containers

• First aid kit for dogs

• Dog booties—made from cordura nylon (useful for protecting worn pads)

• Bags for picking up dog waste

will stress growing bones and joints and may cause irreparable damage. Ask your veterinarian when your dog can backpack safely.

Your vet may want to inoculate your dog against Lyme disease and giardia and start him on heartworm medication, if he is not already on it. You may also wish to discuss tick repellant and a first aid kit for your dog.

Any size dog can backpack, but his usefulness on the hike will depend largely on size. As a rule, you should not have a dog carry more than one-third of his weight without prior conditioning. When starting out, most dogs should carry no more than 20 percent of their weight. For example, a 5-pound terrier shouldn't carry more than a pound (including the backpack) and a 100-pound Malamute should carry no more than 20 pounds. Note that this is a general rule–one pound may be too much for a terrier, so you may have to lessen the weight to just a few ounces. The amount of weight depends on the breed and the dog's condition. If you have any doubts as to whether your dog can carry the weight safely, reduce the weight immediately. Serious injuries can result from too heavy a load.

Purchasing the Right Backpack

A properly fitted backpack is crucial to your dog's comfort. A poorly fitted pack may chafe the dog, bang into his elbows, and decrease the amount of weight he will be able to carry. In extreme circumstances, the pack may chafe so badly it can pull fur out and cause bald spots or may incorrectly place the weight and thereby cause injury.

The pack should rest over the dog's shoulders at the base of the neck and should have a chest strap that clips in front of the dog's chest, as well as a belly band that tightens underneath the ribs. The pack is too small if the bottom of the panniers is more than a couple of inches above the elbows. The pack is too large if the pack extends beyond the hips.

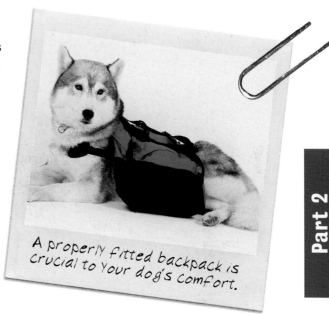

A properly fitted backpack is crucial to your dog's comfort.

Part 2

Extra Features

Other features available with dog packs include:

• Lash panels or D-rings on top. This handy feature allows you to lash coats and other items to the top of the pack.

• Fastex snaps, rather than the old fashion buckles. These snaps are easier to adjust and to fasten and release than the old-style buckles and fasteners.

• Removable panniers. This feature allows you to remove the pack and its contents, while still keeping the pack's base and straps on the dog.

• Curved panniers. Prevents the dog from bumping his elbows into the pack and chafing them or making them sore.

• Ballistic nylon. Packs with ballistic nylon along the bottom of the panniers can take more abuse than packs that have only cordura construction.

• Open mesh on top between panniers. For smaller, lighter packs, open mesh helps dissipate heat. However, the mesh can tear, especially if the dog is carrying heavy loads.

• Reflective tape. Nice for evening hikes or low-light hikes.

• Extra pockets. Always a plus!

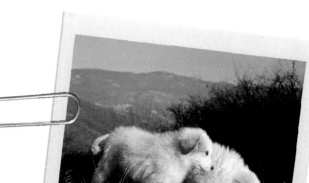

You can start training your dog to backpack while he is still a puppy.

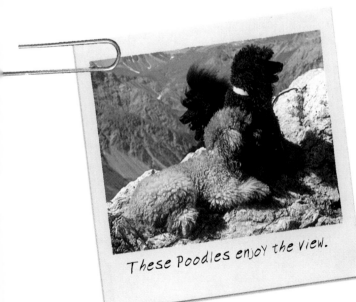

These Poodles enjoy the view.

Introducing the Backpack

Your dog may find the backpack a strange thing indeed when you first strap it on him. Fill the panniers with crumpled newspaper so that he gets used to the extra width when the pack is on. Be certain to give him plenty of praise and treats as you lead him around wearing it. Go for a few walks to get your dog used to the feeling of having it on.

Later, if your dog is over 30 pounds, try adding a soup can in each pannier to add weight. You can slowly add more weight with each session until you've reached 20 percent of your dog's total weight.

How Much Weight and How Far?

Start slowly, hiking with no more than 10 percent of the dog's weight for 2 miles or less. Choose easy terrain. If your dog shows any sign of fatigue, remove the pack and give him water and a rest. As your dog becomes more conditioned to backpacking, try lengthening the hike a mile or so. Vary the terrain. Rough, hilly terrain is harder than flat, compacted trails, so you should shorten the mileage on more difficult hikes. Depending on the breed, dogs can comfortably carry up to 25 percent of their weight over longer distances once they are conditioned. Large, strong breeds, such as Alaskan Malamutes, may be able to carry up to one-third of their weight.

Backpacking Titles

Titles are available either through the national breed clubs or internationally through Canine Backpackers Association (CBA). CBA offers a Pack Dog (PD), Pack Dog Excellent (PDX), Master Pack Dog (MPD), and a Pack Dog Champion (PDCh.) title in three different classes including Alpine, Urban, and Regular. They also offer the option of either Veterans or Juniors.

In order to obtain a CBA Pack Dog (PD) title, the dog must carry 25 percent of his weight on 3 legs of 10 miles each.

In Pack Dog Excellent (PDX), the dog must carry 25 percent of his weight over 3 consecutive days of 10 miles each.

In Master Pack Dog (MPD), the dog must carry 30 percent of his weight over 15 miles. Pack Dog Champions (PDCh.) must earn Masters titles in each of the classes (Regular, Alpine, and Urban) and must hike a total of 500 miles.

Trail Companion titles are similar to pack dog titles, except that there is no mandatory weight requirement.

Part 2

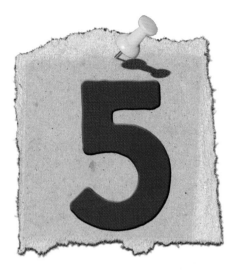

Flyball

Flyball is a fast, competitive sport where teams of four handlers and dogs compete against each other and the clock. The dogs must jump over four hurdles to a flyball box, trigger the box to release the flyball, catch it, and then return over the same hurdles to the finish line and the awaiting relay pair. Teams that complete the relay in under 32 seconds earn points.

The North American Flyball Association (NAFA) sanctions flyball trials and awards titles to flyball participants. Any healthy purebred or mixed breed dog can compete in flyball. Dogs obtain titles based on the number of points earned. The height of the flyball hurdles depends on the smallest canine team member. The hurdles are set 4 inches shorter than

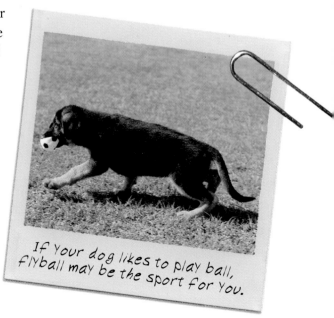

If your dog likes to play ball, flyball may be the sport for you.

the smallest dog on the team (minimum of 8 inches and maximum of 16 inches), so dogs 12 inches and under are usually welcome additions to flyball teams.

Equipment

Flyball requires a flyball box. Plans for constructing one are available in flyball books and on the Internet, or you may purchase a flyball box from an obedience supplier. You will also need four specially constructed flyball hurdles and tennis balls.

How to Train for Flyball

Teaching Your Dog to Catch from the Flyball Box

It helps to have a dog that loves to chase tennis balls. If your dog knows how to play fetch, even better! Teach your dog to catch the ball when you throw it and then call him to you as in a recall. Give the dog praise and treats when he catches the ball and brings it back. Create a command for catching the ball that you will use in flyball. Now, start to throw the ball in the same manner that the ball would fly out of the flyball box.

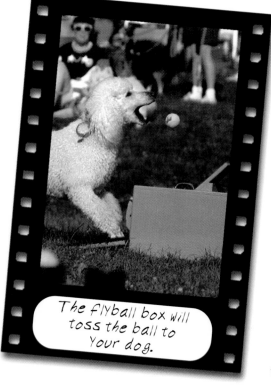

The flyball box will toss the ball to your dog.

Once your dog is proficient at catching the ball, add the flyball box. Step on the flyball box and release a ball. Use the command you have chosen for catching the ball in this new game. It may take a few tries for your dog to catch the ball, but when he knows the catch command, it will be easier. Lavish praise and treats when your dog catches the ball from the flyball box.

Teaching your dog to trigger the flyball box is easy. Take your dog's feet and press them against the flyball box to release the ball. Give your dog the command to catch *before* the ball releases. If your dog is good at it, he may catch the ball as it shoots out. Even if he does not catch the ball, give him a treat and praise for stepping on the box. Keep repeating the action until your dog gets the idea and starts catching the ball.

Teaching Your Dog to Jump

Dogs do not normally know how to jump. Before you begin teaching jumps, make sure that your dog has a clean orthopedic bill of health from your vet. When you start teaching jumps, start as low as you can. If your dog is small, you may want to leave the bar on the ground. Put a leash on his flat collar and lead him to the jump. Carefully lead your dog over it. Use enthusiastic encouragement and the command, "Over!" "Jump!" or "Hup!"

If the jump is on its lowest level, it shouldn't take more than a quick hop to clear it. Give lots of praise and a treat. Many larger dogs will probably walk over it without noticing. This is good–you want your dog to be confident in his approach.

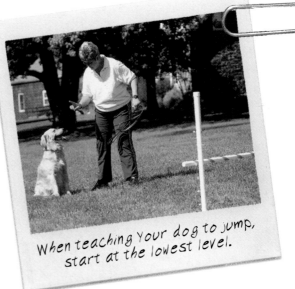

When teaching your dog to jump, start at the lowest level.

Once your dog is completely confident going through the jump, put a long line or tracking lead on his collar. Put him in a sit/stay and walk over to the opposite side of the jump while still holding the leash. Stand on the other side to the right or left of the jump and call your dog over. Gentle tugs and treats in your hand should easily guide him over the jump. Practice directing your dog to the jump from a distance.

Now, raise the bar. It should be at a level where your dog just needs to jump a little to get over it. Practice at the new height until he gets used to it. Then, practice directing him to the jump. Always use treats and praise as a reward. Once your dog is proficient at jumping at a lower height, you can raise the bar and practice at a new height until he is finally at the height he needs to be for competition.

To train your dog to retrieve a tennis ball over the jumps, put a long line on him, toss a tennis ball over the hurdle, have him get it, and then recall him over the jump.

Putting It All Together

Go back to one hurdle and add the flyball box. Give the command, "Over," and then the flyball catch command. Recall your dog over the hurdle, and praise and reward him. If he has learned all the pieces (jumping, pressing the flyball box, and retrieving), this should be easy. If he doesn't complete the command, break down each portion into sections and

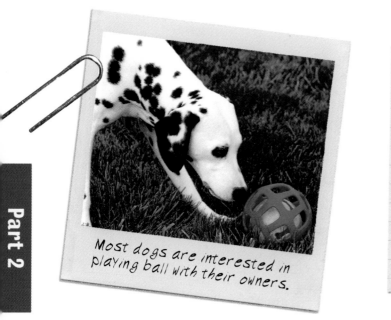

Most dogs are interested in playing ball with their owners.

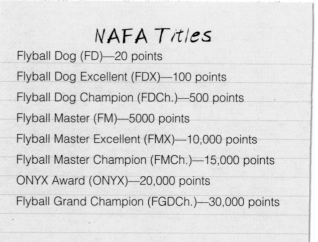

NAFA Titles

Flyball Dog (FD)—20 points

Flyball Dog Excellent (FDX)—100 points

Flyball Dog Champion (FDCh.)—500 points

Flyball Master (FM)—5000 points

Flyball Master Excellent (FMX)—10,000 points

Flyball Master Champion (FMCh.)—15,000 points

ONYX Award (ONYX)—20,000 points

Flyball Grand Champion (FGDCh.)—30,000 points

slowly add each component. Then, as your dog becomes proficient with one jump, add a second jump and send your dog over the hurdles. Eventually, you will have your dog jump all four hurdles to the flyball box and recall over all four.

Flyball Competition

Each team competes against other teams in this fast-paced sport. Dogs on the team earn 1 point for runs under 32 seconds. If the team's aggregate time is under 28 seconds, each dog scores 5 points. If a team is under 24 seconds, each dog earns 25 points.

Dogs earn titles according to the amount of points accumulated.

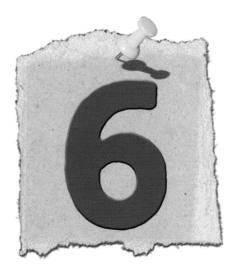

Flying Disc

Playing Frisbee™ or playing catch with a flying disc is so much more fun when you play with your best friend. Your dog probably already knows how to fetch tennis balls and other items, why not add a flying disc to his growing repertoire?

Any healthy dog with good structure, purebred or mixed breed, is eligible to compete in flying disc competitions. Even if you decide not to compete, flying disc is a great way to exercise your dog. Before starting to train for flying disc, inform your veterinarian and have him give your dog a thorough examination. If your dog is a puppy, wait until his growth plates have closed. Ask your vet when your dog can start training for flying disc.

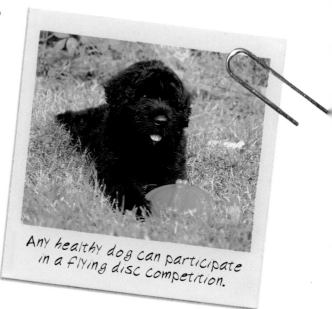

Any healthy dog can participate in a flying disc competition.

Training Your Dog with the Flying Disc

If your dog knows how to play fetch, the flying disc shouldn't be too difficult to teach. Many people start by making the flying disc a desirable object for their dogs. Feed your dog from the flying disc, roll it along the ground on its side so that your dog will chase it, and reward your dog every time he plays with it or picks it up. Some people use a Nylabone FRISBEE® Flying Disc during training, which adds to the interest because they are flavor enhanced. Whichever disc your use, be certain that it is soft and flexible; the hard inflexible discs can hurt or may break teeth.

Choose an enclosed area where your dog can be off leash safely. This is very important, because you do not want your dog to run off while you are training. It is also important to keep distractions down to a minimum. Squirrels, children playing, and other dogs will distract your dog and keep him from learning what you are trying to teach him. Likewise, keep your training sessions short and fun. If your dog is not enjoying the training, stop and do something else that is fun for your dog. Keep the sessions under 15 minutes.

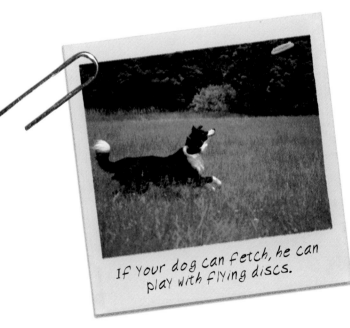

If your dog can fetch, he can play with flying discs.

When you roll the disc, don't allow it to hit your dog. Keep the flying disc a pleasant experience and one that encourages your dog to play with it. When your dog grasps it, give him a command such as, "Take it." Praise your dog if he picks it up. Next, throw the disc near the ground, so that it skims the ground and add the command, "Take it." Give your dog plenty of praise when he chases and catches the disc.

In the meantime, work on your recalls with a long line. A 20- to 30-foot tracking lead or a 20- to 30-foot piece of parachute cord with a snap on one end work well as a long line. Once your dog has mastered recall on command, you can go to the next step.

Next, teach your dog to retrieve the disc. You can do this either with treats or treats and a long line.

Throw or roll the flying disc ten feet away from you and give your dog the command, "Take it." Call him back with your recall command. You may have to tug on the long line to give him the idea or encourage him to come by running backward to get your dog to chase you. If your dog drops the flying disc, pick it up and play with it. Then, run backward, call him, and see if he'll bring it with him. Give him plenty of praise and treats if he returns with it.

You can start teaching your dog to jump for the flying disc as soon as he is old enough to jump. Begin by throwing several easy catches–ones that can be reached by a simple hop. Be aware that dogs can injure themselves by landing wrong, so your flying disc throws should be accurate. Try to throw the disc so that your dog will land straight and on all four feet to reduce chance of injury due to twisting.

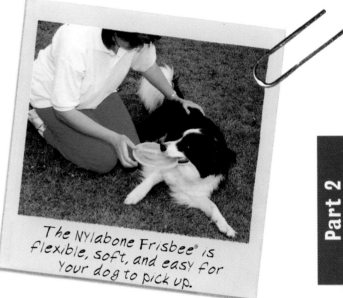

The Nylabone Frisbee® is flexible, soft, and easy for your dog to pick up.

Competition

If you enjoy playing fetch and catch with a flying disc and love showing off, consider trying competition. In competitions, you can show off your dog's talent in one of many different venues of flying disc competition.

Fetch and Catch–The dog and handler must perform as many completed catches as possible in an allotted time.

Freestyle–The dog and handler perform their routine to music.

Accuracy–The handler must throw the flying disc so that the dog will catch the disc within a circle.

Obstacles–The handler must throw the flying disc through or over specific obstacles, and the dog must catch the disc.

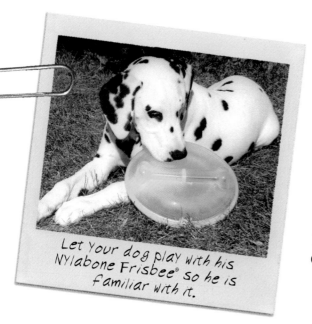

Let your dog play with his NYlabone Frisbee® so he is familiar with it.

Long Distance Events–These may either be done in teams or alone. In the team events, the competition goes for the longest throw/catch, and the team with the short throws is eliminated. Qualifying teams compete against each other and are eliminated until there is a winning team. In solo events, the longest throw/catch wins.

There are both professional and amateur competitions for flying disc events. These events are held both regionally and nationally and include The Flying Disc Dog Open™, ALPO Canine Frisbee™ Disc Championships, and the Quadruped™.

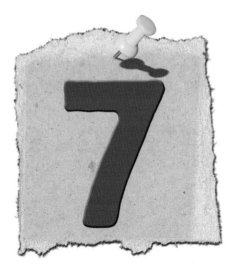

Freestyle Dancing

Do you enjoy dancing, but your friends tend to be all left feet? Maybe your perfect dance partner isn't another human, but your four-footed companion. Freestyle allows you to dance with your dog and have fun. More than just heeling to music, freestyle incorporates a variety of subtle and intricate moves and is fun for both you and your dog.

Freestyle is a relatively new sport that began appearing in the 1990s. The very first freestyle routine was developed by Val Culpin in British Columbia, Canada, and was performed by Dawn Jecs and her Border Collie, Checkers, in 1989. In 1991, Musical Canine Sports International (MCSI) was founded in Canada, with Ventre Advertising (Patti Ventre) as its

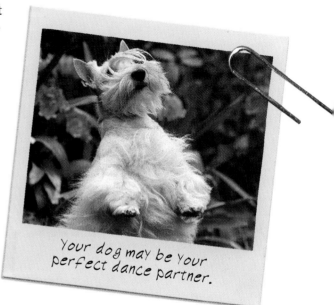

Your dog may be your perfect dance partner.

promoter. The beginnings of the World Canine Freestyle Organization (WCFO) evolved from this union with Patti Ventre as promoter and president. MCSI eventually evolved into WCFO. Officially, WCFO was founded in June 1999. Another organization, Canine Freestyle Federation (CFF), holds events as well.

Any dog, purebred or mixed breed, may participate in freestyle competitions. You can have multiple dogs and partners, or you may dance with just one dog. Creativity is paramount in freestyle dancing.

How to Get Started
Freestyle Formats

Freestyle has two basic formats: Heelwork to Music and Musical Freestyle. Each format may be split into classes: Juniors, Singles, Pairs, and Teams.

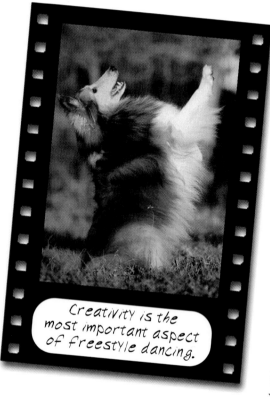

Creativity is the most important aspect of freestyle dancing.

Heelwork to Music requires that the dog stay within 4 feet of the handler at all times. The dog may not perform any distance work. This includes jumps, weaves, send outs, distance spins, and pivots. Props are allowed, provided that they are part of the routine in some fashion. Training collars of any type, other than a standard slip collar, are not allowed, nor are training aids (food, toys, etc).

Musical Freestyle has fewer rules than Heelwork to Music. Any move, provided it is not dangerous, may be used. Innovation and creativity are the keys here. Props are allowed, provided that they are part of the routine in some fashion. Training collars of any type are not allowed, nor are training aids (food, toys, etc.).

Proficiency Tests

WCFO offers a variety of proficiency tests for those

interested in Musical Freestyle and Heelwork to Music. The proficiency tests are required to earn Dancing Dog titles. The proficiency tests are ranked as follows:

Bronze Bar

Bronze Medal

Silver Bar

Silver Medal

Gold Bar

Gold Medal

Each proficiency test requires that the dog perform a certain number of maneuvers. The number of maneuvers and their difficulty increases with each subsequent test.

For example, you do not need to be a WCFO member to take the Bronze Bar Proficiency Test. The test may either be done live or videotaped. If videotaped, the videotape may not be edited in any way, and there must be a witness affidavit. Although the number of moves are limited, these tests are very difficult and require a certain sequence of movement. The required moves include:

Right About Turn;

Left About Turn;

Backing;

Speed Changes;

Circle in Heel Position.

The Bronze Medal Heelwork to Music is the next proficiency test after the Bronze Bar.

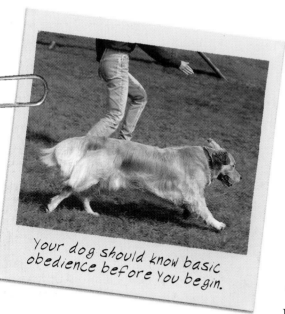

Your dog should know basic obedience before you begin.

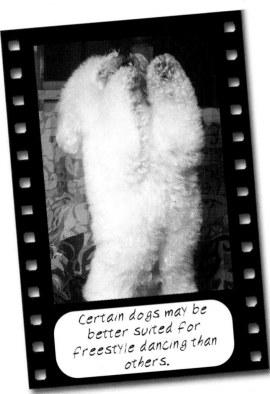

Certain dogs may be better suited for freestyle dancing than others.

Although the number of moves is limited, these tests are very difficult and require a certain sequence of movements. The required moves include:

Right about/left about turns moving forward;

Heeling on right moving forward minimum 10 steps;

Backing up in heel position 10 steps;

Side pass in front position minimum of 6 steps;

Simultaneous spins by dog and handler.

Training for Freestyle

Before you begin teaching your dog his freestyle moves, listen to different music to determine what fits your style and your dog's style. Start playing with your dog while listening to the music–you'll get a good feel for what suits your dog's temperament and gait.

Order some freestyle videos from either WCFO or CFF so you are able to watch how it's done. Their moves will give you ideas for training your dog, as well as choreography and costumes.

Your dog should know heel, sit, down, stay, front, stand, back up, and other obedience commands. These commands will make up the backbone of the freestyle routine. Other moves such as pivots, circles, and serpentines are not obedience commands, but an owner can quickly teach them using positive reinforcement techniques.

Begin teaching your dog to heel on both sides, since

heeling is required on the right and left sides. An owner can teach quick front and turns using food as a reward for the correct behavior. You can teach a dog to back up by moving forward with a slack leash and either gently crowding the dog backward or holding a tidbit overhead and slowly moving it just behind the dog's head and out of reach.

Even if you never compete or win a title, the fun you'll have dancing with your dog will be worth the time and effort.

Part 2

Teaching Tricks

Trick training can be fun for both you and your dog. Many dogs love doing tricks because of the extra attention and praise they receive. You'll enjoy it because you can show off your talented dog and impress your friends. Some tricks, such as fetch, ring a bell, and go find, can actually be useful. You can teach your dog to find a missing item or to ring a bell when he needs to go outside.

Not all dogs have the temperament for performing tricks. If trainability is a concern, try the most instinctive tricks such as shake hands or speak. (Fetch is not instinctive to all breeds–you'll have good luck with retriever breeds and breeds known for trainability). If your dog seems to enjoy these tricks,

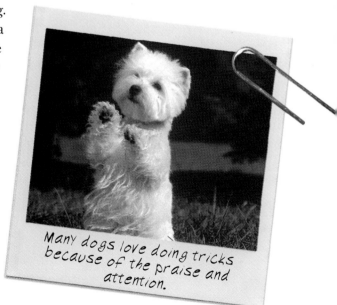

Many dogs love doing tricks because of the praise and attention.

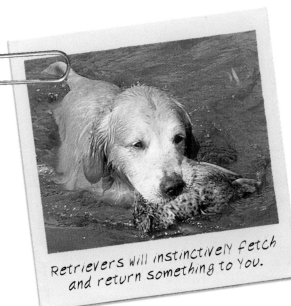

Retrievers will instinctively fetch and return something to You.

try others. You may be able to make up some new tricks with your dog.

The "trick" to teaching tricks is to make the training as fun as possible. Don't spend hours training. Instead, try a few short sessions while playing with your dog. It will make learning more fun.

Fetch

The desire to fetch is not instinctive in all dogs. Nevertheless, you can teach your dog to fetch while playing. If your dog has a favorite toy, play with him and his toy for a while. Then, take the toy and toss it a few feet away. Many dogs will chase something that is thrown. If your dog chases the toy and picks it up, try to get him to return with the toy. Praise and reward him with a treat. Toss it again and see if he'll carry it back. Use the command, "Fetch!" as you toss it so that he associates the action with the command.

Some dogs will run over to the toy, some will ignore it, and others will pick it up only to drop it when you call them to you. If your dog is one that ignores the toy, try smearing peanut butter or something tasty on it and offer it to him. Then, take it and toss it a few feet. If it's really tasty, your dog will go after it. Praise him and offer to trade a treat as a reward.

If your dog still doesn't look at the toy, find a toy that will interest him or use a clicker to create interest. Usually, smearing the toy with peanut butter or beef juice works. To get your dog to bring the toy back, throw it a very short distance–maybe a few feet away or, if that is too far, right in front of your dog. Once he picks it up, call him to you and offer a treat as a trade. With each successful retrieve, offer praise and a treat. When he is confident with this exercise, increase the distance a tiny bit and repeat the exercise.

It usually doesn't take long to teach a dog fetch. Often, it becomes the dog's favorite game and can be the precursor to teaching your dog to compete in more complicated activities, such as hunting tests or field trials.

Shake Hands

Shake hands is very natural for many dogs if they paw their humans. Place your dog in a sit. Gently take his paw in your hand and shake it. Say, "Shake" or "Paw." Follow this by "Good dog!" and a treat. After a few times, your dog will be ready to offer his paw to get the praise and the treat!

Speak or Bark on Command

This is a little more difficult than teaching your dog to shake hands. First, your dog must be somewhat vocal. When you hear him bark, say, "Speak!" and praise him. Sometimes giving a treat will enforce barking on command. It takes a few times, but most dogs will learn that "Speak!" means bark.

Beg or Dance

This should only be taught to dogs that do not have hip or back problems. Command your dog to sit and then offer a treat just above his nose. When he rises to try to grab the treat, say, "Beg!" and release the treat as a reward. Increase the height so that your dog has to reach a little more each time. Release the treat when your dog has achieved the height–soon he may be on his hind legs!

Once your dog has become proficient at the beg command, you may wish to try the dance command. You can teach your dog to dance by moving the treat in a circle away from him. Start only with a few inches. Your dog will try to reach the treat by turning around. Give him the treat and praise. Start by saying, "Beg!" and then "Dance!" As you increase the circle, your dog may be soon doing pirouettes!

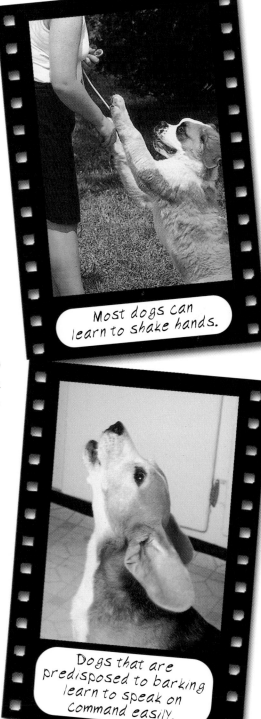

Most dogs can learn to shake hands.

Dogs that are predisposed to barking learn to speak on command easily.

Part 2

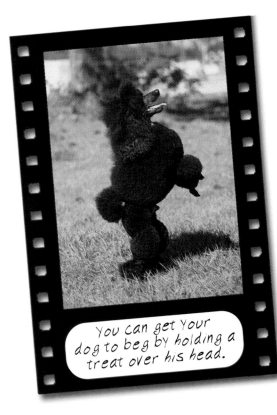

You can get your dog to beg by holding a treat over his head.

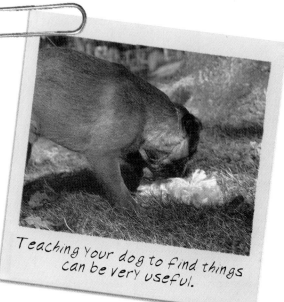

Teaching your dog to find things can be very useful.

Go Find

"Go find" is a useful command, particularly for people who often lose or drop things. You should work on one item first. Start by getting your dog interested in the object. (You can do this with a toy or something such as keys.) Using a clicker will help facilitate the interest. When your dog touches or shows interest in the object, tell him, "Keys!" or whatever the object's name is, and give him a treat. You may need to put something tasty on the object. (Note: Don't do this with something fragile or something that will be stained.)

Once your dog touches the object, give the command, hide it in clear view, and let him search for it. For example, say, "Keys!" and praise him and give him a treat when he finds them. After he has mastered finding the item, hide it by partially covering it with a newspaper (let him see you prepare this). Again, give him the command, "Keys!" and let him find them. If he has trouble with this, lead him to the object and help him discover it. Do this several times until he learns to look for the item beneath stuff, not just on top.

Work toward full concealment. Eventually, your dog will even find something completely buried under the newspaper. You can use the "Go find" command with people, too. For example, have your dog "find" your child by having the child hold a treat. Give the command, "Go find Johnny!" as your child calls your dog and offers him a treat.

Ring a Bell

This trick can be useful when your dog needs to go outside. Hang a bell next to the door where your dog goes out. When you are ready to let him out, take his nose and hold it against the bells so that they ring. Then, praise him and let him out.

After a few rounds of this, your dog will nose the bells all by himself to alert you that he needs to go out.

The tricks that you can teach your dog are only limited by your imagination and your dog's enthusiasm and can provide entertainment for the entire family.

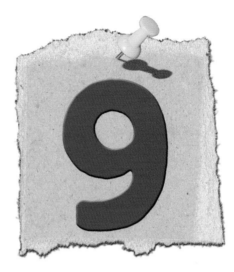

Therapy Dogs

Part 2

Therapy dogs provide positive support for patients in hospitals, at nursing homes, and at other care facilities. A pet's healing effects are well known to the many volunteers who bring their dogs to these facilities. Dogs often can help withdrawn patients become less reclusive and more cooperative. Patients enjoy their nonjudgmental manner and frequently form special friendships with therapy dogs.

Training for Therapy Dog Work

Therapy dogs do not require any special training beyond good manners and general obedience training. Temperament is important, and your dog should become used to having strange people pet and touch him. Some organizations, such as

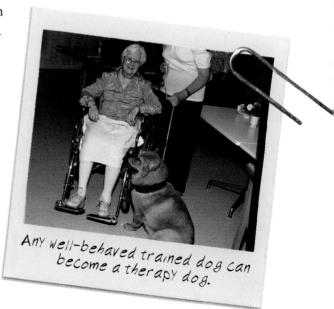

Any well-behaved trained dog can become a therapy dog.

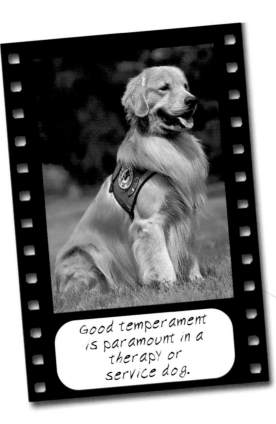

Good temperament is paramount in a therapy or service dog.

Eligible Breeds

Any well-behaved dog may become a therapy dog, regardless of breed or size. Mixed breed or purebred dogs are welcome to become part of the program. The dog should have obedience training and pass a Canine Good Citizen® or other temperament test. Tricks aren't necessary, but many therapy dogs know how to "speak" or "shake hands" on command. Most important are the dog's personality, temperament, and obedience.

Therapy Dog International and Delta Society Pet Partners®, require that your dog pass a modified version of the AKC Canine Good Citizen® (CGC®) test. Delta Society Pet Partners® also require that prospective therapy dog owners attend a workshop or complete the at-home version of the Pet Partners Team Training Course, which requires a further aptitude test.

Titles

Dogs that work as therapy dogs are certified under the organization they are registered with, but do not have official titles. These dogs do earn temperament test titles such as CGC®, among others. Contact the therapy organization for a list of titles, if applicable.

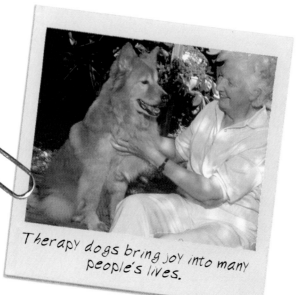

Therapy dogs bring joy into many people's lives.

Therapy Dog Training

You can contact the following organizations for information or contact a local hospital or nursing home in your area to find out how to get involved locally.

Delta Society
289 Perimeter Road East
Renton, WA 98055-1329
(425) 226-7357 (8:30 a.m. - 5:00 p.m. PST, Monday - Friday)
(425) 235-1076 (fax)
www.deltasociety.org
info@deltasociety.org

Therapy Dogs International, Inc.
Attn: New Registrations
88 Bartley Road
Flanders, NJ 07836
(973) 252-9800
(973) 252-7171 (fax)
www.tdi-dog.org
tdi@gti.net

Part 2

Part Three
Getting More Competitive

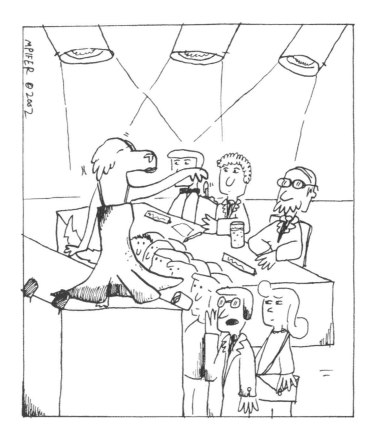

"I've heard about dog shows being competitive, but this is ridiculous!"

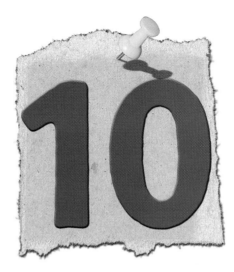

10

The Canine Good Citizen® Test

In 1989, the American Kennel Club started the Canine Good Citizen® (CGC®) program to recognize dogs that have good manners both at home and in the community. Unlike other AKC titles, the Canine Good Citizen® title is available to all dogs, purebred or mixed breed, at any age. Technically, the CGC® is not an official AKC title; however, dog owners may put the CGC® designation after their dog's names.

The CGC® was created to provide a means of encouraging responsible dog ownership. The series of tests are as follows:

Accepting a Friendly Stranger–The dog must show no fear when a stranger approaches his owner

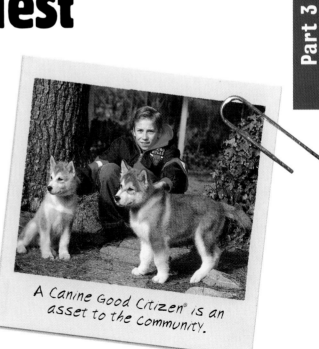

A Canine Good Citizen® is an asset to the community.

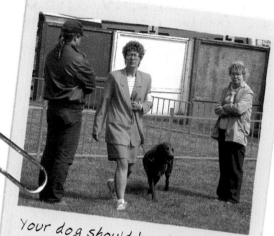

Your dog should be able to walk nicely beside you on his leash.

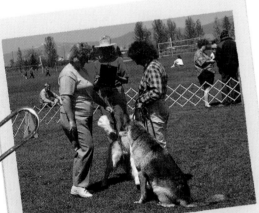

Getting along with other dogs is part of the Canine Good Citizen® test.

and talks to him or her.

Sitting Politely for Petting–The dog must accept petting by a stranger when he is with his owner.

Appearance and Grooming–The dog must accept being brushed gently by the evaluator and allow the evaluator to pick up each foot and examine his ears. The evaluator also judges if the dog is clean and groomed.

Walking on a Loose Lead–The dog must walk on a loose lead with the handler, including turns and stops.

Walking Through a Crowd–The dog must walk through a crowd of people without pulling, jumping on people, or acting fearful.

Sit and Down on Command/Staying in Place–The dog must sit and lie down on command. The dog must then stay in place while the owner walks 20 feet away and returns to him. The dog may change position, but must stay in the same place.

Coming When Called–The dog must wait while the owner walks ten feet and then calls the dog. The dog must come to the owner.

Reaction to Another Dog–The dog must show no more than a casual interest in another dog as that dog and handler approach the first dog and owner.

Reaction to Distraction–The dog must show no fear when faced with two everyday distractions. The dog may show curiosity but not aggression or shyness.

Supervised Separation—The dog must accept being left with the evaluator for three minutes while the owner is out of sight.

Training for the CGC® Exercises

The CGC® test is a basic temperament and obedience test. Before taking the test, your dog should know how to walk nicely on a leash, and the sit, down, come, and stay commands. If your dog has any difficulty with any of these commands, review them so that he is reliable while on leash.

The best way to train for the temperament test portions is to start socializing your dog. Socialization should starts when your dog is a puppy. He is ready to meet the world after he has had his last series of vaccinations—usually after 16 weeks. Before this time, you run the risk of exposing your pup to deadly diseases.

You need to bring your dog to different places and allow him to meet strangers. Training classes, fun matches, and dog parks are great ways to socialize your dog. Some

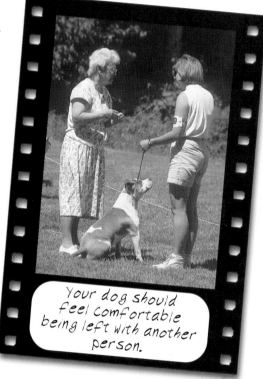

Your dog should feel comfortable being left with another person.

owners bring their dogs to supermarkets and stand outside, allowing them to experience crowds of people and frequent petting. Bringing your dog to parks and other places where people and pets gather is a great way to get your dog used to distractions.

Ask some friends to meet with you and your dog in a neutral place—a park or other public place where pets are allowed. If, at any time, your dog becomes fearful or shy, reduce the contact a bit until he becomes comfortable. For example, if your dog is shy when several of your friends try to pet him, don't insist it. Instead, allow your dog to walk on leash with your friends nearby or have just one person pet him.

Never correct a dog for shyness—this leads to more negative behavior. Instead, try distracting your dog with food or by lessening the encounter. If your dog is excited and boisterous, correction is all right, provided it is appropriate. Use the sit or down command and act deliberately calm so that your dog will settle down as well. Being in a hurry tends to aggravate excited dogs, so move slowly and don't rush. If your dog becomes wild with

Part 3

A canine good citizen makes a great neighbor and family pet.

excitement, try using a crate or practicing a long down in a quiet place until he settles down.

Each positive encounter helps to socialize your dog. It's a lesson that will stay with him throughout his life. The key to training is to be calm and deliberate when performing these exercises. If you are nervous or worried, you will telegraph these feelings to your dog.

If your dog is aggressive toward other people or other dogs, consult a professional dog trainer or behaviorist. The CGC® test is designed to prove that the dog is a model canine citizen. The test will not make your dog a less aggressive dog. You should first correct any problems associated with aggression before trying to obtain a CGC®.

Part 3

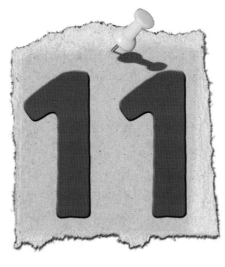

Agility

Ever since agility wowed audiences at the Crufts Dog Show in England in 1978, it has taken off as one of the fastest growing dog sports. Agility, in its simplest form, is a fast-paced sport where dogs jump over hurdles, go through tunnels, and climb on dog walks, over teeter-totters, and up A-frames set out in a particular course. The run is timed and the dog that makes the fewest mistakes in the least amount of time wins. The handler shows the dog where to go using signals and commands. Agility is great fun for both people and dogs.

Unlike obedience, which requires repetition, agility courses are constantly changing. Dogs that may not do well in obedience often enjoy agility. It takes

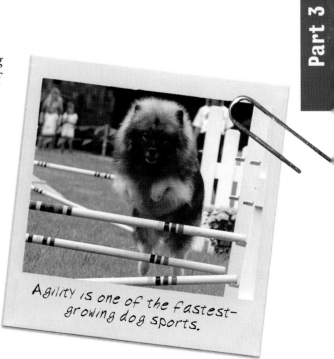

Agility is one of the fastest-growing dog sports.

Types of Agility

Agility is a relatively new sport, but there are plenty of agility associations with their own "brand" of agility. The following is a list of agility sanctioning bodies in the United States and Canada:

AKC (American Kennel Club)—AKC offers a variety of titles in both Standard Class and Jumpers with Weaves. Only purebred dogs either with regular registration or an ILP (indefinite listing privilege) registration may enter. ILP dogs must be neutered.

NADAC (North American Dog Agility Council)—NADAC offers a faster version of agility based on British rules. It offers Juniors and Veterans classes, as well as Standard, Jumpers, and Gamblers courses. All dogs are allowed: purebred or mixed breed.

UKC (United Kennel Club)—UKC offers a version of agility based on control and preciseness. It offers Agility I, Agility II, and Agility III courses. UKC equipment varies considerably from AKC, NADAC, and USDAA in their Agility II division. All dogs are allowed to compete with UKC registration, provided mixed breeds are neutered.

USDAA (United States Dog Agility Association)—USDAA offers a faster version of agility based on British rules. It offers Standard, Jumpers, Relay, and Gamblers courses. It offers a champion program and a slower performance program, as well as a Junior Handler class. All dogs are allowed to compete: purebred or mixed breed.

ASCA (Australian Shepherd Club of America)—ASCA follows NADAC rules. ASCA and NADAC often offer combined trials. Competition is open to all dogs—not just Australian Shepherds.

AAC (Agility Association of Canada)—AAC is an agility organization within Canada only.

a short time to master the obstacles, but it takes a long time to perfect handling and sequencing.

Agility is highly competitive. Each year, national agility associations hold their competition to determine which dogs are the very best. Agility is not just for purebred dogs. While AKC only allows purebreds in competition, United States Dog Agility Association (USDAA), North American Dog Agility Council (NADAC), and United Kennel Club (UKC) all allow mixed breeds to compete for titles. Nor is agility only for the able-bodied. UKC has special concessions for handicapped handlers. All you need is a healthy dog.

Preparing for the Competitive Agility Trial

At some point in agility, you will start thinking about competition. Even people who are in agility "just for fun" eventually become addicts and attend their first trial. But before you enter your dog, be certain that he is properly trained. Knowing the obstacles is not enough. Many novices have learned how difficult and frustrating an agility trial can be because both they and their dogs were ill prepared.

Luckily, many agility clubs hold fun matches. You can get a taste for competition, while at the same time, provide a valuable training experience for both you and your dog. Ask the judge beforehand if it is all right if you do some training in the ring. Tell them that you do not intend to compete for anything and are just looking for the experience. Most judges will be open to this.

Be certain that your dog is reliable off-leash. Many agility trials and fun matches are held outdoors. If your dog is not reliable off-leash, consider only entering indoor trials and matches until he is reliable. Agility trial premium lists state whether the trial is held indoors or out.

How do you locate an agility trial in your area? Contact the local agility clubs or, if you do not know of any, contact the national agility organizations for lists of clubs and trials in your area. Some organizations are widespread throughout the United States; others are fairly regional. Request a premium list from the trial secretary and find out the entry deadline. In some locations, the trial actually fills up before the deadline.

What class should you enter? If this is your first time in agility, you'll enter a Novice class, usually called Novice or Starters. There may be sections in the Novice class, usually called A and B. Novice A is for those handlers who have never owned a dog with an agility title. This way, Novice A people do not have to compete with Novice B people for placements.

With all the major agility organizations, there are multiple styles or types of agility. AKC recognizes

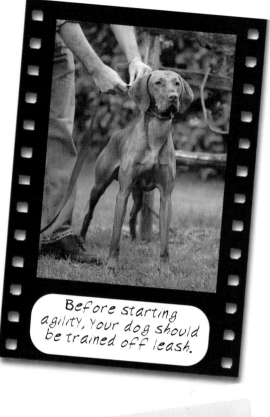

Before starting agility, your dog should be trained off leash.

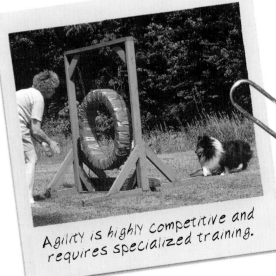

Agility is highly competitive and requires specialized training.

Part 3

Agility Classes

Not surprisingly, your dog can earn various titles within agility—even within one organization! Your dog can compete in fun agility courses that offer variety and challenges to both the handler and dog.

Standard Class (All organizations)—The Standard Class is a normal agility course, complete with contact obstacles, jumps, and other obstacles recognized by the organization.

Jumpers Class (NADAC and USDAA)/Jumpers with Weaves (AKC)—The Jumpers Class offers a course that contains only hurdles and tunnels. (In Jumpers with Weaves, these include weave poles.) It is faster than the Standard Class.

Gamblers Class (NADAC and USDAA)—The course is laid out in sequences. A point value is assigned to each obstacle. The handler and dog are then given a certain amount of time to accumulate points and may choose whichever obstacles they wish. After the point accumulation phase ends, the whistles blows and the handler and dog are required to perform a "gamble," that is, a sequence of obstacles that the judge has assigned. To make this more challenging, the handler must stay a certain distance away from the dog.

Relay Class (USDAA)—This requires two or four teams of handlers and dogs. The handler and dog pair must complete the course and "pass the baton" to the next member of the team. The fastest team wins.

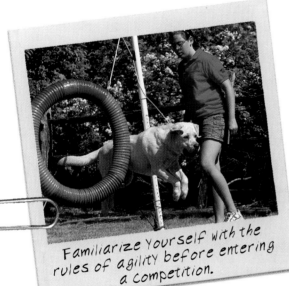

Familiarize yourself with the rules of agility before entering a competition.

Standard and Jumpers with Weaves. USDAA recognizes Standard, Jumpers, Relay, and Gamblers. NADAC offers Standard, Jumpers, and Gamblers. UKC offers AG-I and AG-II. If you are not familiar with these classes, stick with Standard (AG-I) and watch the other classes to see how they are run. The variety in agility is what makes such a fun sport.

The Competitive Trial

Going to your first trial can be daunting. There are many dogs, loud noises, crowds, and interesting smells. If you can, arrive early so that your dog can become accustomed to the sights and sounds of the trial. You may receive the running order list and a number as a confirmation in the mail before the trial. Some organizations do not provide this; in this case,

Part 3

check the judging program for the running order. Most programs have check-in times.

Familiarize yourself with the agility trial regulations for the organization holding the event you plan to enter. If you aren't certain what a rule means, consult an experienced agility competitor or judge. Most are happy to explain the rule in that particular organization.

Check In

When you first arrive at a trial, you will want to check in with the stewards. These people will assign you a number and possibly a tag with your number on it to wear in the ring. Some trials provide course maps for you to study.

Trials usually run from most experienced (Excellent Classes) to least experienced (Novice) and from the shortest height to the tallest height. Many reverse it the next day, but do not count on this. Always ask what the running order is and keep track of it throughout the day. You will have time to watch other classes and socialize.

Locate a quiet place to set up your crate and your equipment. Many clubs set aside crating areas, but often the crating area is limited and very crowded. This is why it is important to show up early.

The judge's briefing, walkthrough, and contact familiarization (if performed) may occur in any order (at the judge's discretion), so pay attention

Items to Bring to a Trial

Trials are typically held in parks, at fairgrounds, and in horse arenas. They may be held at any time of the year. You should consider the weather and location when packing items. Although larger trials may have vendors for food and drink, expect to bring your own. Here is a partial list of items you may want to bring:

√ Water for both you and your dog

√ Water bowls

√ Crate for your dog (exercise pens work well too)

√ Leash

√ Collar (if collars are allowed)

√ Treats for your dog

√ Snacks for you

√ Plastic mat or ground cover to keep dirt off you and your dog

√ Folding chair

√ Reading material or other entertainment for yourself

√ Toys for your dog

√ Tent or awning if outdoors

√ Portable fans (if summer)

√ Raingear or poncho

√ Warm clothing

√ Hat for sun

√ Sunglasses and sunblock

√ Cash (for vendors/food)

Part 3

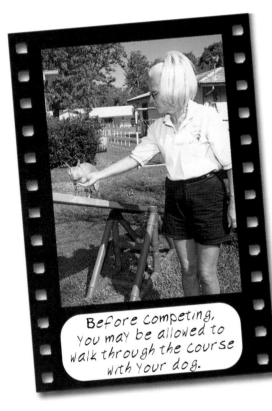

Before competing, you may be allowed to walk through the course with your dog.

to when your Novice Class is about to start. Do not miss any of these, as they will help you prepare for your run-through.

The Judge's Briefing

The judges briefing is where the judge introduces himself or herself and tells you what to expect from his or her judging. If a table is employed, the judge will tell you whether a sit or down needs to be performed and will perform the count so you will know how long it is. The judge may go over hand signals or other potential signals (such as the whistle), and will give the course times.

Now is the time to ask questions! If you have a particular question concerning the course, ask the judge. He or she should be happy to answer any questions you may have.

The Walkthrough

All organizations have a walkthrough. The walkthrough is where you familiarize yourself with the course without your dog. The walkthrough will determine how you will handle your dog during your run-through.

You cannot bring toys or food with you inside the ring, so empty your pockets, and crate your dog while you familiarize yourself with the course. If you have a question regarding the equipment's safety or placement, ask now.

Contact Familiarization and Course Familiarization

AKC allows contact familiarization, that is, a chance for your dog to perform the contact obstacles (seesaw, A-frame, and dog walk) once to get your dog used to this type of surface. In UKC, the dog actually performs a *course* familiarization. In the course familiarization, the dog takes each obstacle in the course one time.

The Run-Through

The run-through takes less than two minutes. Arrive early at the entrance to the ring. Tell the gate stewards you are there; otherwise, they may assume you are absent and may not

Part 3

call your number. You may not have treats, toys, or any training device when you enter the ring. Your dog may not wear a collar in USDAA trials and may not wear a training collar in NADAC, AKC, or UKC trials.

You must start your dog behind the starting line, usually marked by two orange cones. If your dog crosses that line any time after the timers say they are ready, your time starts. Likewise, the timers do not stop the clock until after your dog crosses the finish line. So, be certain you know where both lines are.

You cannot touch your dog while you are running the course. If you accidentally touch or bump your dog in the correct direction, you may be disqualified. You may not use harsh commands or be threatening or abusive to your dog in any way. The judge will be looking for missed contacts (dog fails to touch a contact area), refusals (AKC only– where the dog passes or balks at the obstacle instead of performing it), off-courses (the dog takes the wrong obstacle or takes the obstacle in the wrong direction), fly-offs, and other ways to fail to perform.

The goal is to have a clean run; that is, no errors and under time. However, as a beginner, your goal should be to have a good time with your dog. Watch the judge for points lost.

After you get through the course, praise your dog. You want him to feel as if he were the best dog on the course, regardless of his actual performance.

If your dog has qualified (or in NADAC, even if he

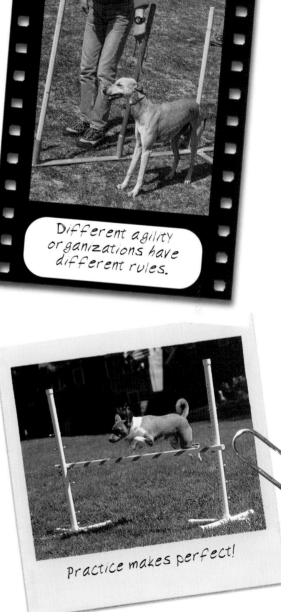

Different agility organizations have different rules.

Practice makes perfect!

Part 3

Agility Trainers

You may want to get professional help with training your dog for agility competitions. The following are some guidelines to help you choose the best trainer for you and your dog. Ask these questions:

• Is the trainer familiar with agility? Is he familiar with the style of agility you want to train in? If he's not, look for a trainer who is. Inexperienced trainers can inadvertently cause problems by using the wrong training methods.

• Does the trainer train you to train your dog? You are the other half of the team. If you do not know the correct way to handle your dog, your dog's training is useless to you.

• Does the trainer use positive methods to train dogs? Agility should only use positive methods.

• Does the trainer have references?

• Does the trainer own dogs with agility titles? Does he compete for titles? The trainer should be familiar enough with agility to have put agility titles on his or her own dogs.

• Does the trainer allow you to watch a training session? There are no "training secrets." If the trainer is afraid that you will "steal his secrets," look elsewhere. He should have nothing to hide.

• Is the trainer gentle or harsh with dogs? The trainer should be positive toward the dogs—firm, but gentle.

• Does the trainer's philosophy coincide with your own? This is a matter of personal taste.

• Do you like the trainer? You will not learn from someone whom you dislike.

• Does the trainer have equipment that is regulation standard? Your dog should train on regulation-sized equipment. Otherwise, when you attend a trial, your dog may experience difficulties with the equipment.

• Does the trainer have enough room for run-throughs or at least sequencing? Only part of agility training is equipment training. The trainer should have enough room for sequencing (three or four obstacles in a pattern) or for a trial run-through.

• Does the trainer work on obstacles and sequencing? The trainer should teach *both* obstacles and sequencing.

• Does the trainer have a regimented class or is it a drop-in type class? Both are useful, but the novice should look for a regimented class and then use drop-in classes to refine techniques.

hasn't), he may be in the running for a placement. Wait for the announcement of scores and times to find out if your dog has placed in his height division and class.

Agility Obstacles

Introducing the obstacles correctly will make agility more fun and easier to train your dog. Look for an introductory class that will help teach your dog the obstacles or look for a drop-in class that will let you work on a particular obstacle until your dog gets it right.

Agility is best taught using positive reinforcement methods. This includes finding a motivational object, such as food or a toy. Use that motivational object as a reward for your dog. Because it is fun, it takes very little time for agility itself to become the motivation. Many dogs love agility and that becomes its own reward.

Do not rush through the obstacles. A negative encounter with an obstacle may dampen your dog's enthusiasm for the sport. Start slowly and don't rush through teaching them. What appears easy for you is complex and new for your dog.

When you start out, you will want to use a leash for training. Some facilities allow training collars; others do not. Keep your dog on a leash until he is comfortable with all of the obstacles and is reliable off-leash. USDAA requires that the dog "runs naked," that is, without a collar. UKC requires a dog to wear a collar, but without tags. AKC and NADAC allow collars, but require that the collars have no tags. Training collars are not allowed in trial runs.

The following are "standard" obstacles that you will see in most forms of agility. Other nonstandard obstacles do appear, but if your dog has mastered these obstacles, it doesn't take long to learn the new ones.

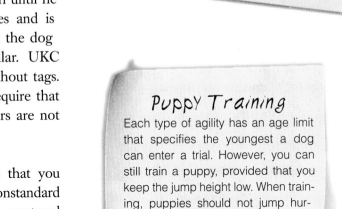

This mixed breed flies over the hurdles.

Puppy Training

Each type of agility has an age limit that specifies the youngest a dog can enter a trial. However, you can still train a puppy, provided that you keep the jump height low. When training, puppies should not jump hurdles higher than their hock height until the puppy is full-grown. Ask your veterinarian when it is safe to jump your dog.

Part 3

Hurdles

Hurdles or jumps are one of the most common obstacles your dog will encounter. They can be with or without "wings"; that is, decorative panels on each side of the jump. Spread hurdles require the dog to jump two or three bars. A broad jump requires the dog to clear several boards lying on the ground.

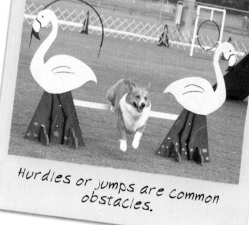

Hurdles or jumps are common obstacles.

The height at which the jumps are set depends on the height of your dog at the shoulder. All agility competitions have different jump heights.

Start teaching your dog to jump by setting the hurdles at the lowest height. If your dog would normally jump 8 or 12 inches in competition, lay the bar on the ground. Use a leash and lead your dog over the jump. Give a command such as "Over," "Hup," or "Jump." Offer treats to lure your dog over and give him treats and praise when he performs the jump correctly.

As your dog becomes used to this height, increase the difficulty by one jump height and practice that. If your dog is small, that jump may be at or close to competition height. If your dog is a large breed and must jump over 20 inches, increase the jump to 16 inches or so and practice there.

Gradually move the bar up to full competition height. Your dog should learn what full competition height is like, but you should train at lower heights to avoid injuring your dog's legs. Use practice run-throughs at full height, but keep general practice jumps lower.

Tire Jump

The tire jump is a hurdle with a tire or black irrigation hose in the form of a circle that the dog must jump through. It is the most technically demanding of the jumps because the dog often does not see it as a jump. Instead, the dog may try to walk underneath the tire. The tire's height is measured from the ground to the inside diameter of the tire. It is set at the same height as other hurdles.

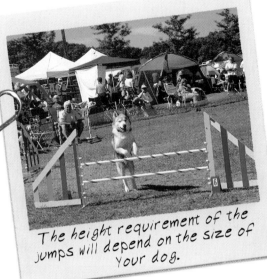

The height requirement of the jumps will depend on the size of your dog.

Train for the tire jump as you would any other hurdle. Use treats to lure your dog through the jump and praise him when he jumps through. If he tries to climb underneath the tire, try putting a board or another jump in the open space below the tire. You may use the same command as other hurdles or may use a separate command such as "Tire" to differentiate it from other jumps.

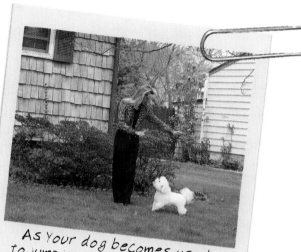

As your dog becomes used to jumping, gradually increase the height.

A-Frame

The A-frame, the seesaw, and the dog walk make up the "contact obstacles." These are called contact obstacles because the dog must walk across them and must touch contact zones to perform the obstacle correctly.

The A-frame is a large contact obstacle that has two 8- to 9-foot ramps that meet at a peak in the center. The ramps are 3 to 4 feet wide. The dog must climb the A-frame to the top and then scramble down the other side.

Lower the A-frame if the training center allows you to do so. This will make it less intimidating. Otherwise, you may have to train at full height. Use a command such as "Frame" or "Scramble" and lead your dog over the A-frame. If your dog is nervous, keep his leash tight in one hand and a treat in the other. Try to keep him focused on the treat as you lead him across.

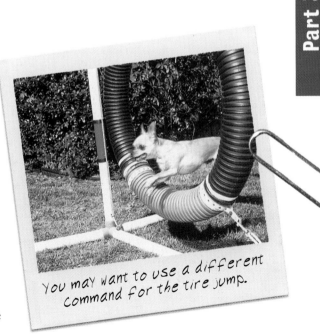

You may want to use a different command for the tire jump.

After the next few times on the A-frame, your dog may climb it without encouragement. Teach him to pause on the yellow contact surface using the command "Wait" or "Rest." To do this, slow your dog as he approaches the

Part 3

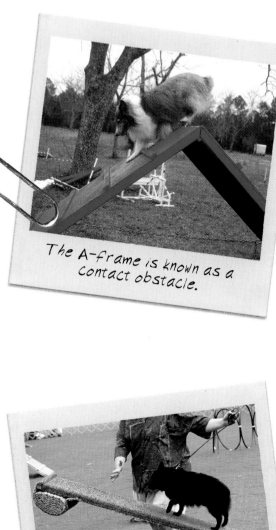

The A-frame is known as a contact obstacle.

Your dog must touch the entry and the exit of the seesaw to complete the obstacle.

downward contact and command him to sit when he touches the contact portion.

Once your dog is comfortable with the lower height, raise the A-frame to the competition height. Practice at this new height several times to have your dog become accustomed to it.

Seesaw

The seesaw or teeter-totter is similar to the children's playground equipment but without handles. The dog must enter the seesaw at the downward end, walk across it until he tips the plank, and then walk down the plank. This obstacle can be intimidating to new agility dogs because it moves with the dog's weight. If the dog is unprepared for the seesaw to tip, it can crash down with a loud bang, scaring the dog. Like the A-frame, the seesaw has contact patches that the dog must touch on both the entry and exit of the seesaw.

Wait until your dog is comfortable with other obstacles before attempting the seesaw. You will need a second person to help steady the seesaw while you lead your dog over. Give your dog the command "Teeter" or "Seesaw" and lead your dog over the seesaw, using treats. Stop your dog before the tipping point and say, "Tip it." You and the second person should hold the other side of the teeter so that your dog does not slam it down. As you move your dog forward, let the seesaw tip gently until the end touches the ground. Do not allow the seesaw to bang or it may spook your dog.

If your dog becomes fearful, stop everything and give him some time to calm down. Praise him and give him treats, and then start again. It may take a few times before your dog learns to tip the seesaw properly. Don't allow him to rush off the teeter once he tips it. Instead, put him in a sit on the contact area with a "Wait" or "Rest" and then give the release signal.

Dog Walk

The dog walk is a tall obstacle that has two narrow ramps joined by a long plank. The dog must walk up the narrow ramp while touching the contacts, cross the long plank, and then walk down the other ramp, touching the contacts. There are two sizes to the dog walk– one with 8-foot long planks and the other with 12-foot planks. The 12-foot dog walk is much taller than the 8-foot variety.

Lead your dog up the ramp, focusing his attention on the treat rather than the obstacle. Lead him across the walk portion, then down the ramp, stopping at the contact patches with a "Rest" or "Wait."

Large dogs may find the dog walk intimidating, so another method of training the dog walk is called *backchaining*. In backchaining, the owner sets the dog on the downward ramp and walks the dog off. The owner then sets the dog a few feet farther up the ramp and walks the dog off. After the dog becomes comfortable with the new position, the owner moves the dog back a foot or so and begins the process again. In this way, the dog learns that in order to leave the obstacle, he must walk forward to walk off.

Pipe Tunnel

The pipe tunnel or open tunnel is a favorite obstacle for most dogs. The tunnel is a large pipe with a 24-inch width diameter that can flex into different shapes. The dog must enter the pipe tunnel, run through it, and then exit it.

Straighten the pipe tunnel and then push it together so that it is only a few feet long. Have someone hold your dog while you thread his

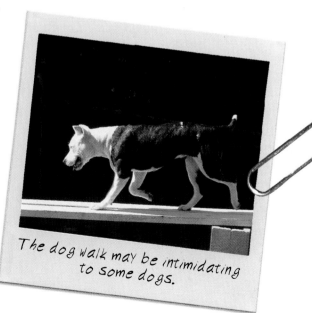

The dog walk may be intimidating to some dogs.

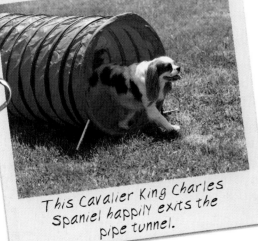

This Cavalier King Charles Spaniel happily exits the pipe tunnel.

leash through the tunnel to the other side. Kneel at the other side of the tunnel, while holding your dog's leash. Call him through the tunnel. You may need to lure him with treats and praise.

Practice the tunnel in this configuration a few times until your dog becomes used to it. Use the command, "Tunnel," or another word that you will use to uniquely describe the tunnel. Then, lengthen the tunnel a bit and practice with it in the new configuration until your dog becomes comfortable with it. Continue to lengthen the tunnel until your dog is confidently going through while it is fully extended and straight.

At this point, add a small bend to the tunnel. Some dogs have no difficulty with not seeing the other side; others will refuse to go in. If your dog is nervous about entering what appears to be a closed tunnel, make the bend in it less severe so that he may see a little of the other side. As he becomes more confident with the tunnel, increase the bend. Eventually, your dog should be able to enter a tunnel in a horseshoe configuration.

Closed Tunnel

The closed tunnel, collapsed tunnel, or chute starts with a ridged, circular opening. It is connected to a chute constructed from parachute material that the dog must push through to complete the obstacle. Many dogs new to agility find the chute daunting at first because it appears to go nowhere. Dogs can accidentally become tangled in the chute, so it is very important to make certain it stays flat.

Like the seesaw, this obstacle should be one of the last obstacles to be taught. Your dog may find the closed tunnel disconcerting because he will have to push his way through the fabric. Start by rolling up the chute material and having someone hold your dog while you kneel at the other end. Hold the chute material open so that your dog can see you and the exit. Call your dog through. If your dog has learned the pipe tunnel, this new tunnel should not be any concern. Use the word "chute" or another word to uniquely describe this obstacle. Some people use the same word, "tunnel," for both the pipe tunnel and the closed tunnel, only to find a pipe tunnel and a closed tunnel side-by-side on a trial course!

Once your dog is confident with the closed tunnel in this configuration, lengthen the chute material and allow a little sag in it. Call your dog. He should walk straight through. Lower the chute a little at a time, allowing your dog to push through the material. Eventually, you will be calling your dog through the closed tunnel in its final configuration.

Pause Table

The pause table is an obstacle that looks like a square table. It is set to the height of the jumps. The dog must jump onto the table and perform a sit or down on command and remain there for a count of five.

Most dogs are used to jumping up on things (your dog may be allowed on furniture). In this case, the table is not a difficult obstacle. However, teaching your dog to stay on the table for a count of five may be more difficult. Start by luring your dog onto the table and then trying the sit or down for five seconds.

Weave Poles

The weave poles are possibly the most difficult obstacle to master. They are PVC poles that are arranged in a straight line that your dog must weave through. Weaving is not intuitive to a dog–it must be learned.

A popular method of teaching weaves is *channeling*. This requires either stick-in-the-ground weave poles or special training weave poles that will create a channel. The weave poles are arranged in two columns separated by a distance equal to the dog's shoulder width. Put your dog on a leash and have him

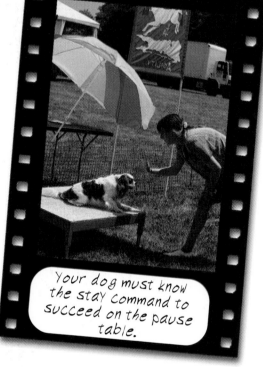

Your dog must know the stay command to succeed on the pause table.

Organization-specific equipment

There are other types of equipment that not all styles of agility recognize. These include:

• Sway bridge—a suspension bridge that sways when a dog crosses it.

• Swing plank—a plank that is suspended at the four corners; it moves when the dog crosses it.

• Wishing well jump—a jump that looks like a wishing well.

• Window jump—a jump shaped like an open window.

• Cross-over—a tower-like structure that has four planks that meet in the center.

• Tower—a structure that has a plank, stairs, and slide.

• Pause box—a square made from PVC that lies on the ground; the dog must treat it like a pause table.

• Platform jump—the dog must climb on the box, sit, jump over the hurdle, and then sit again.

• Crawl tunnel—a type of tunnel the dog must crawl underneath.

• Hoop tunnel—a type of "open" tunnel the dog must go through.

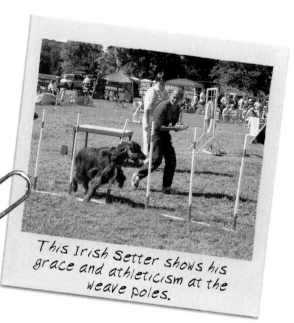

This Irish Setter shows his grace and athleticism at the weave poles.

run through the two columns for two weeks. Then, move the weave poles one inch closer to each other. Now the dog will have to bend to move around the columns. Practice in that configuration for two more weeks. Then, move the poles in an inch and continue to practice that way for two more weeks. Eventually, the poles will be moved into a single column, and your dog will weave properly.

Part 3

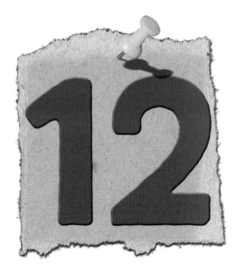

12

Obedience

Every dog needs to learn obedience commands, regardless of whether the dog is a pet, a working dog, or an obedience trial champion. Obedience training focuses the dog on his owner and helps channel excess energy. Obedience-trained dogs make better pets. They're more enjoyable to have around, and trained dogs are happy dogs

Basic obedience includes walking on leash without pulling and obeying the sit, down, stay, and come commands. Most dog owners start teaching their dogs these basic commands when their dogs are puppies. Perhaps your dog knows sit and come already.

At six months to one year, you should enroll in an

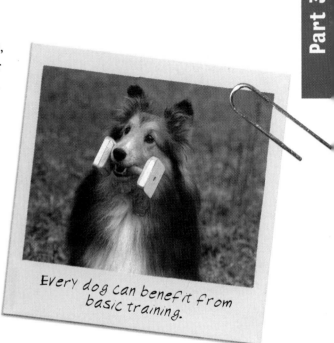

Every dog can benefit from basic training.

Types of Leashes and Collars

Without the correct leash and collar, training can become very difficult. When training your dog, you should use a six-foot leather leash and a slip or training collar. These provide the most control when training. Other types of collars and leashes include:

• Flat, buckle, or rolled collar—Use for identification. Attach your dog's tags to this. Some trainers recommend a flat or buckle collar for training, as well.

• Halter collars—Actually, these are head halters designed to stop dogs from pulling. They may restrict breathing and in certain conditions may cause overheating.

• Prong collars—These collars are used for strong pullers. Never leave a dog wearing a prong collar unattended. Do not use these collars in place of flat collars for everyday wear.

• Slip collars—Commonly called "choke chains," these collars are not intended to choke the dog. They are standard training collars. Never leave a dog wearing a slip collar unattended. Do not use these collars in place of flat collars for everyday wear.

• Tracking leads—These leashes are useful for distance work with your dog.

• Flexible leads—These leashes are useful to teach the come command, but provide no control and may break if snagged. Do not use them with strong dogs or when hiking.

• Leather leads—These leashes provide the most control, as well as the most comfort for your hands.

• Nylon leads—These leashes will often cut into your hands and provide little control.

• Chain leads—These leashes offer no control and are poor choices for training.

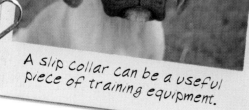

A slip collar can be a useful piece of training equipment.

obedience class. Choose one with a professional trainer experienced in working with your breed; otherwise, you may be wasting your money. Discount trainers are usually not a bargain when it comes to certain breeds such as hounds or Northern breeds, as many have not had experience training these creative and stubborn dogs. As said before, look for a trainer who teaches *you* to train your dog and one that uses a combination of positive reinforcement techniques.

Practice with your dog for 10 minutes per session every day. Your dog will enjoy the interaction and the time spent with you, and you will have a better behaved pet.

Basic Commands

Sit

You can easily teach your dog to sit. Start by holding a treat just above your dog's nose. Bring the treat backward while gently pushing down on your dog's rear end and give him the command, "Sit!" When your dog sits, give him the treat and praise him.

Walking on Leash and Heeling

Start by teaching your dog to sit by your left side. Lure the dog into a proper sit and then give him a treat. You should have a large amount of treats in your pocket. Break biscuits into little pieces or use tiny puppy treats, otherwise you will have a very fat dog by the end of training!

Clip the leash onto your dog's training collar and command, "Heel." Hold a treat in your hand as you both start walking–let him see that treat. Your dog should be focused on your hand and not on forging ahead.

When your dog is at the right speed, neither lagging nor pulling, offer him the treat and praise him. If he forges ahead, use the collar and treat to lure him back to the proper position and praise him again. When you stop, put your dog in a sit and give him the treat. In this way, through positive reinforcement, you can train your dog to walk nicely on lead.

Down

Once you teach your dog the sit command, you should teach him the down. Start by placing him into a sit, and attach a leash to his collar. Take a treat and lower it from nose level to the floor, while gently pulling downward on

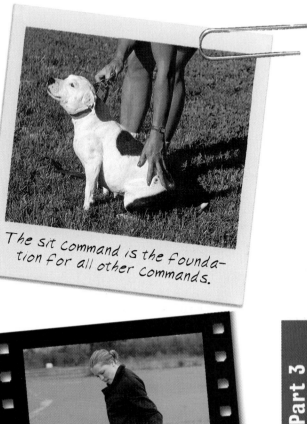

The sit command is the foundation for all other commands.

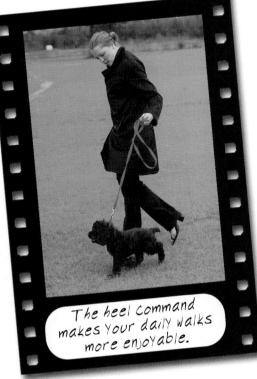

The heel command makes your daily walks more enjoyable.

Part 3

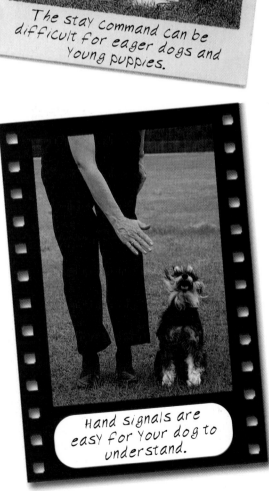

The stay command can be difficult for eager dogs and young puppies.

Hand signals are easy for your dog to understand.

the collar. Give your dog the command, "Down!" You can also help him by gently taking his front legs and lowering him into a down. Give him a treat and praise him each time.

Stay

Once your dog has learned sit and down, he should learn the stay command. Put him in a sit beside you while on leash. Tell him, "Stay!" and use a flat open hand in front of his face for emphasis. Take a step or two away from him and then turn to face him. If he tries to move, tell him, "No! Stay!" and put him back into position. It usually takes a few times for the dog to learn that you want him to remain in position. Keep him in the stay for 10 seconds. Return to him, release him with the command, "Okay," and then praise him and offer him a treat.

Practice the stay in both sit and down. You will slowly lengthen the amount of time or the distance of the stay, but not both. If your dog breaks during the stay, decrease the amount of time or distance. Only increase the distance or time again when your dog is staying reliably.

Come

Start by attaching a six-foot leash onto your dog's collar. Put him in a sit/stay and walk out to the length of the leash. With a treat in one hand, call your dog, "Fido, come!" If he does not come, show him the treat and gently reel him in. When he arrives, give him the treat and praise him. Practice this several times each day.

You can train your dog to come longer distances using a long line or retractable lead. Follow the same procedure as you did using the six-foot leash. If your dog does not come immediately, start the exercise over and use a shorter distance next time. Always offer a treat when your dog comes back to you regardless of whether you had to use the lead or the dog returned voluntarily.

Off-lead recalls are tricky with certain breeds. Some dogs, such as sighthounds and Northern breeds, usually take much more time to be reliable off leash. Never let any dog off leash unless that dog has been trained to be reliable. Practice in a fenced-in area where your dog cannot escape.

To begin training the come command, have a favorite treat or toy and put your dog in a sit/stay. Start from six feet away and call your dog to you, giving him the treat or toy when he comes. If he does not come or dashes away, do not chase him. Lure him over with treats or quickly walk in the opposite direction. Most dogs will come around to see what you are doing and then you can catch them. When you do catch your dog, do not yell or punish him. You should always praise and reward him for coming to you. Then, practice recalls on leash for another two weeks.

Do not train in an open area where your dog can get away from you. You might be able to train your dog to be reliable on off-leash recalls, but only after long, consistent training. Even then, it takes only one opportunity for a dog to escape.

Competitive Obedience

Competitive obedience was developed to demonstrate a dog's ability to behave properly at home and in public places. The first AKC obedience trial was held in 1933. Obedience trials were patterned after trials held in England.

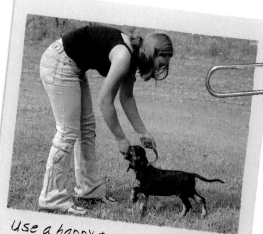

Use a happy tone of voice when you call your dog to you.

Part 3

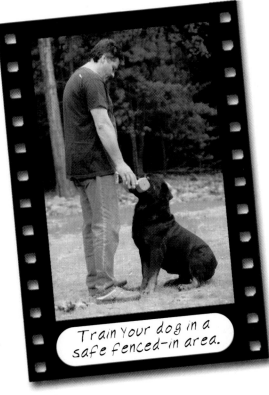

Train your dog in a safe fenced-in area.

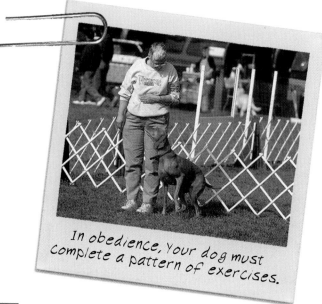

In obedience, your dog must complete a pattern of exercises.

In competitive obedience, the dog must complete a series of exercises. For example, for the Novice title, the dog must heel on leash, off leash, heel in a figure eight, stand for examination, come when called (the recall), and perform a long down and sit. It sounds easy, but given the rigorous requirements, it can be very challenging for some dogs and owners.

Both the AKC and the UKC offer obedience titles to purebred dogs. The UKC offers titles to mixed breed dogs as well. Their program is similar to AKC's, but check UKC rules for variations.

Companion Dog

A dog earns the Companion Dog (CD) title having achieved three qualifying legs in the Novice Class. The maximum number is 200, with a minimum qualifying score of 170. In addition, a dog must earn more than 50 percent of the points for each exercise. A dog may compete in Novice A or Novice B. Novice A is for dogs with owners that have never earned an obedience title before. Novice B is for dogs with owners that have previously earned at least one obedience title.

A Novice dog must perform the following exercises to obtain a qualifying score:

Heel on leash and figure eight–40 points

Stand for examination–30 points

Heel free–40 points

Recall–30 points

Long sit–30 points

Long down–30 points

Companion Dog Excellent

A dog earns the Companion Dog Excellent (CDX) title after earning a CD and then earning three qualifying legs in the Open Class. The maximum number of points is 200, with a minimum qualifying score of 170. A dog may compete in either Open A or Open B. Open A is for dogs with owners that have never earned an OTCh. (Obedience Trial Champion) before. Open B is for dogs with owners that have earned OTCh. titles on their dogs. Dogs may continue to compete in Open B after they have earned a CDX.

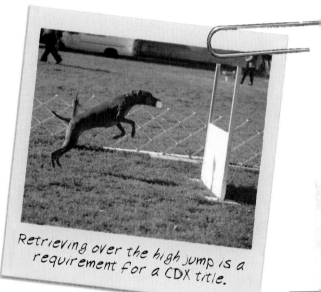

Retrieving over the high jump is a requirement for a CDX title.

An Open A dog must perform the following exercises to obtain a qualifying score:

Heel free and figure eight–40 points

Drop on recall–30 points

Retrieve on flat–20 points

Retrieve over high jump–30 points

Broad jump–20 points

Long sit–30 points

Long down–30 points

Open B dogs must perform the same exercises, but they may be performed in a different order, depending on the judge's decision.

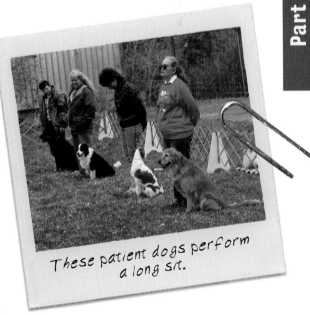

These patient dogs perform a long sit.

Utility Dog

A dog earns the Utility Dog (UD) title after earning a CDX

and then earning three qualifying legs in the Utility Class. The maximum number of points is 200, with a minimum qualifying score of 170 and more than 50 percent of each exercise. A dog may compete in Utility A or Utility B. Utility A is for dogs with owners that have never earned an OTCh. before. Utility B is for dogs with owners that have previously earned OTCh. titles.

A Utility A dog must perform the following exercises to obtain a qualifying score:

Signal exercise–40 points

Scent discrimination Article #1–30 points

Scent discrimination Article #2–30 points

Directed retrieve–30 points

Moving stand and examination–30 points

Directed jumping–40 points

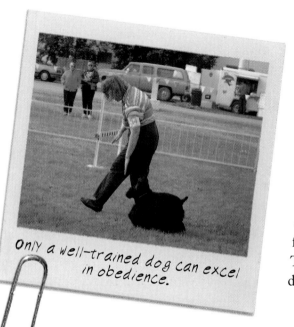

Only a well-trained dog can excel in obedience.

Utility B dogs must perform the same exercises, but they may be performed in a different order, depending on the judge's decision.

Obedience Trial Champion

A dog earns his Obedience Trial Champion (OTCh.) title after having earned a UD and 100 points in Open B and Utility B, and 3 first-place wins (1 in Open B, 1 in Utility B, and 1 in either) under 3 different judges with 6 or more dogs competing. Points are accumulated by winning first through fourth place in the above classes. The number of points depends on the number of dogs competing.

Utility Dog Excellent

The Utility Dog Excellent (UDX) title requires a UD and then earning qualifying legs in the Utility B and Open B Classes in ten separate trials.

Training for Novice—Earning a CD Title

Training for competitive obedience is quite different from basic obedience training. Competitive obedience requires the dog to follow the commands precisely. You cannot repeat the command without penalty, and, in many instances, you cannot combine a command with a hand signal unless the particular exercise stipulates "command and/or signal."

The best way to learn these exercises is to attend a professional obedience class. Here, you will find trainers who are familiar with obedience competition and can best teach you how to train for it. Some trainers are actually obedience judges and can help you prepare for a trial.

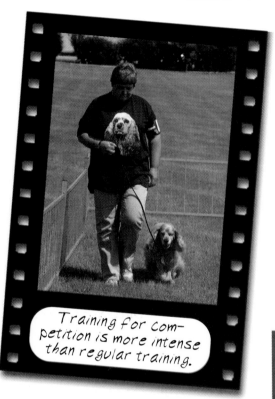

Training for competition is more intense than regular training.

The Heel Position

A dog that has had any obedience training should already know the heel position. If not, teach that now. The correct position for heel, sit, and down is on your left-hand side, facing forward. This is known as the heel position. When walking your dog, you should have your left hand holding the leash loosely to control the dog and any excess leash looped in your right hand. This will give you the maximum control over a dog–even a large or strong one.

When teaching the heel position, move your dog to your left side. After he stands or sits for a few moments in heel position, give him a treat and praise him. Use a one-word command such as "Place" or "Heel" to indicate the heel position. Practice putting your dog in the heel position and reward him when he stands or sits straight in that position. Do not reward a sloppy performance. Try again and give your dog the treat when he is in the proper position.

Heel on Leash

In the heel on leash exercise, you will follow the judge's commands. The judge will ask if you are ready and then say, "Forward." He will then issue orders in any sequence to observe how well your dog heels and how you work as a team. These include:

Halt–The handler must stop and the dog must sit straight in the heel position.

Forward–Go forward in a straight line.

Right turn–The handler and dog must turn right.

Left turn–The handler and dog must turn left.

About turn–The handler and dog must turn around and continue in the opposite direction.

Normal–The handler and dog must resume their regular pace.

Slow–The handler and dog must slow their pace to less than normal.

Fast–The handler must run, and the dog must accelerate appreciably to maintain the heel position.

Start by training your dog to heel in the proper position. When you stop, you may need to give the sit command so that your dog will sit each time you stop. Begin by having your dog sit beside you in the heel position with training collar and leash on.

Hold a treat in your left hand. Give the command, "Fido, heel!" and start walking, left foot first. If your dog starts to forge ahead or lag behind, get his attention by showing him the treat and lure him into the correct position. When he is in the correct position, praise him and give him a treat. If your dog is unsure and lags, pat your leg and encourage him to come beside you. Likewise, if he forges ahead, pull back on the leash or lure him back with a treat. Give him the treat when he is in the proper position.

When you stop, have your dog sit in the heel position and give him a treat. When you start again, always start with the left foot first. Dogs see the left leg movement before the right leg moves. Also, it becomes another signal to your dog that he is to move with you.

Figure Eights

Figure eights require that the dog heel with the owner around two stewards who stand eight feet apart. The dog and handler stand midway between the stewards facing the judge. The judge asks if the handler is ready and then gives the handler the command, "Forward." The handler and dog must walk in a figure-eight pattern without the dog lagging or sniffing. Unlike the heel on leash, there are no other commands, except forward and halt. The dog must sit when the handler halts.

Figure eights are tricky because the handler cannot adapt his pace to the dog's pace or he will receive a nonqualifying score. Likewise, the handler cannot jerk the dog forward. When training for figure eights, the handler needs to encourage the dog around the training pylon and slow down for the straight sections. In this way, the dog learns to maintain one speed at all times.

Stand for Examination

The stand for examination requires the handler to remove the leash from the dog and hand it to the steward. The judge orders the handler to: "Stand your dog for examination and leave when you are ready." The handler puts the dog in heel position and then stands the dog. The handler then gives the dog a stay command, turns and walks six feet away from the dog, turns to face the dog, and then waits for judge to examine the dog. The judge approaches from the front, allowing the dog to sniff the hand. The judge then touches the head, body, and hindquarters of the dog. The judge then gives the command, "Back to your dog." The handler must walk all the way around the dog to return to the heel position. The dog may not move until the judge gives the command, "Exercise finished."

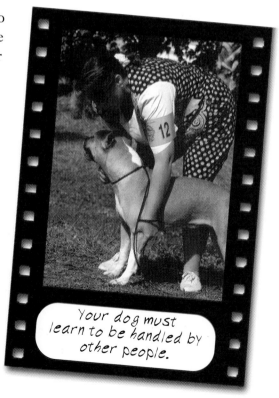

Your dog must learn to be handled by other people.

This is a tricky exercise, as dogs cannot move their feet without points being deducted. A dog that moves out of place, sits, or lies down earns a

Part 3

nonqualifying score. Shyness or reluctance to being touched can also cause points to be deducted.

If your dog does not know the stay command, begin teaching this now. Once your dog has mastered the heel position and the stay, put your dog in a heel position and use a treat to lure him into the stand position. Use the command, "Stand." When your dog does this, even for a second, give him a treat.

Once your dog learns the stand command, begin teaching him the stay command. Do not leave his side at this time. Let him stay for a few seconds and then release him with the okay command. If he breaks his stay, put him back into the exact stay position. As he becomes more confident in his stand/stays, lengthen the amount of time he needs to hold that stay.

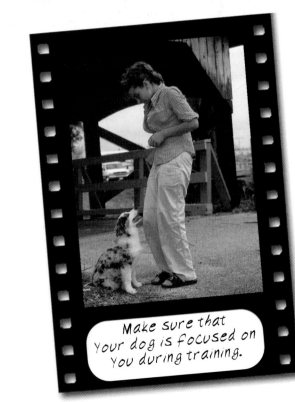

Make sure that your dog is focused on you during training.

To add a new element, stand your dog, give him a stay command, and then take a couple of steps and turn around. Leave with the right foot this time–the left foot is the signal to heel. If your dog moves forward, move him back to the heel position and give him another stay command. If your dog makes a habit of breaking the stays, shorten the stays or the distance between you and him until he is reliable.

The Recall
In the recall, the handler sits his dog and gives him the command, "Stay." The judge gives the order, "Leave your dog." The handler must then walk to the end of the ring and turn around. The judge will then give the order, "Call your dog." The handler must call the dog. The dog must come in a straight line and sit in front of the handler. The judge will then give the command, "Finish." The dog performs a finish; that is, either goes around the handler or turns around in place to be in the heel position.

If your dog does not know the come or stay commands, work on these first. When you begin teaching the recall, your may wish to hold a treat in your mouth or use your hands to bring your dog to a perfect sit in front of you. You will not be able to do this in the ring, so do not allow your dog to depend on your hands being used as a signal.

Finishing your dog is more difficult. Start by using a treat to lure your dog into the correct position while using the command, "Place," "Heel," or "Finish." When your dog follows the treat correctly, give it to him and praise him.

Heel Off Leash

The heel off leash is the same as the heel on leash but with the dog off leash. The judge's orders are the same as they are for heel on leash.

Do not attempt to work your dog off leash until his on-leash heeling is perfect. Use treats as you would to keep your dog focused on heeling, rather than being off leash. When you start working off leash, have your dog on a leash and a light parachute cord or fishing line with a small snap at the end. Remove the leash, but keep the line on your dog as you heel. Do not use the line unless your dog tries to bolt.

Long Sit

Both the long sit and the long down are performed as group exercises. After the recall, the handler must wait until there are enough handler/dog pairs to be divided into equal sections. The handlers must line their dogs up in the order that they appear in the catalogue at the trial. The judge will

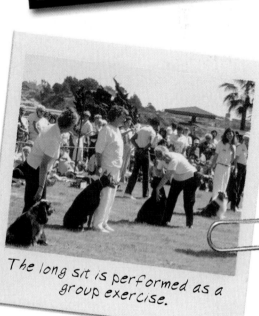

Heeling off leash is part of an obedience trial.

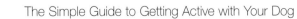

The long sit is performed as a group exercise.

Part 3

tell the handlers, "Sit your dogs" and then, "Leave your dogs." The handlers may give a stay command and then must walk to the other side of the ring and stand facing their dogs. Dogs must stay in the long sit without moving, whining, or barking. After one minute, the judge will tell the handlers, "Return to your dogs." At that time, the handlers must walk around their own dogs to the heel position. The dog cannot move from the sit during this time until the judge says, "Exercise finished."

When you start teaching the long sit, build up to longer times but stay at a short distance from your dog initially. As your dog becomes comfortable, gradually lengthen the distance between you and your dog.

Long Down

After the long sit, the judge will tell the handlers, "Down your dogs" and then, "Leave your dogs." The handlers must give the down command and leave their dogs. The handlers may give a stay command. The handlers must then walk to the other side of the ring and stand facing their dogs. Dogs must stay in the long down without moving, whining, or barking. After three minutes, the judge will tell the handlers "Return to your dogs." At that time, the handlers must walk around their own dog to the heel position. The dog cannot move from the down during this time until the judge says, "Exercise finished."

When you start teaching the long down, gradually lengthen the time, but stay a short distance from your dog initially. As your dog becomes comfortable, gradually lengthen the distance as well as the time.

Preparing for Competition

Once you and your dog have learned the exercises for Novice, you should practice these exercises both at an obedience training facility and at home. Some dogs do well practicing every day, others require time off.

Many local clubs hold fun matches that include obedience. These fun matches allow you to practice with your dog and have the experience of being in the

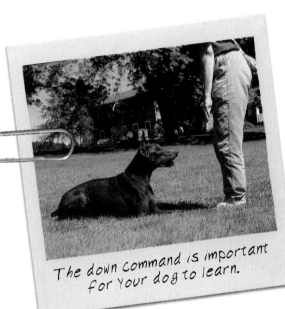

The down command is important for your dog to learn.

ring without being in an actual trial. Some sanctioned matches may not allow training in the ring, but fun matches usually do. If this is your first time at a fun match, let the judge know. If you are training in the ring, you may not place in the class, but since this is only for fun, you should not be competitive. Enjoy yourself and use this match to train and see how well your dog is doing.

Your First Trial

Obedience trials are often held in conjunction with conformation shows, but some are held separately. If you do not know where these shows are, contact a local obedience training facility or club or talk to people who show their dogs in conformation. They should be able to tell you who to contact regarding local shows. You can also contact AKC or UKC directly to find out who superintends the shows in your area. Once you obtain the contact information, request the lists for upcoming shows.

Be certain that your dog is reliable off leash, unless he is entered in Novice classes at matches. In Pre-Novice, the dog must stay on leash the entire time. Pre-Novice is considered a precursor to training for Novice. Many obedience trials and fun matches are held outdoors. If your dog is not reliable off leash, consider only entering indoor trials and matches until he is reliable. Obedience trial premium lists state whether the trial is indoors or out.

What class should you enter? If this is your first time in competitive obedience, you'll want to enter Novice A. There is a differentiation in the Novice class between A and B. As mentioned before, Novice A is for those handlers who never owned a dog with an obedience title.

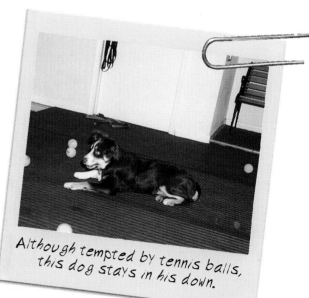

Although tempted by tennis balls, this dog stays in his down.

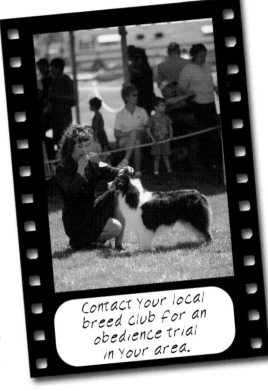

Contact your local breed club for an obedience trial in your area.

What to Bring to an Obedience Trial

Trials are typically held in parks, at fairgrounds, and in horse arenas. They may be held at any time of the year. You should consider the weather and location when packing items. Although larger trials may have vendors for food and drink, expect to bring your own. Here is a partial list of things you may want to bring:

√ Water for both you and your dog

√ Water bowls

√ Crate (exercise pens work well, too)

√ Leash

√ Treats for your dog

√ Plastic mat or ground cover to keep dirt off you and your dog

√ Folding chair

√ Reading material or other entertainment for yourself

√ Toys for your dog

√ Tent or awning

√ Portable fans

√ Raingear or poncho

√ Warm clothing

√ Hat for sun

√ Sunglasses and sunblock

√ Cash

Going to your first trial can be daunting. There are many dogs, loud noises, crowds, and interesting smells. Both you and your dog may find the whole trial distracting. If you can, arrive early so that your dog can become accustomed to the sights and sounds of the trial. You may receive the catalogue order list and a number as a conformation in the mail before the trial.

Checking In

When you arrive at the trial, you will want to check in with the steward in your and pick up your armband. Locate the ring early–trial rings are often not the easiest to find, especially if there is a conformation show held in conjunction.

Even though trials with over 30 entries must post times for each class, you may or may not know the exact time you will be in the ring. This depends largely on the number of entrants ahead. Many judges may move faster or slower, and participants could be caught unaware. If you have a conflict (such as having another dog in a ring about the same time), notify the stewards immediately. They will work with you to resolve the conflict.

Once you find your ring, locate a quiet place to set up your crate and your equipment. This

Part 3

is not always an easy task at trials held in conjunction with conformation shows! Many clubs set aside crating areas, but these are often very crowded, so get there early.

Your Turn in the Ring

Your turn in the ring for the individual exercises takes less than two minutes. Arrive early at the entrance to the ring. Tell the ring stewards that you are there; otherwise, they may assume you are absent and may not call your number. You may not have treats, toys, or any training device when you enter the ring. The judge will ask you if you have any questions when you enter the ring. Use this opportunity to ask any pertinent questions or to indicate any problems you might have hearing commands. Most judges are helpful.

Although it is normal to be nervous in the obedience ring, try to relax and have fun. Once you are done with your individual exercises, wait for the group exercises. Most judges have their own way of handling dogs that break a long sit or long down–do what the judge tells you to do.

Once the long down is complete, praise your dog. Praise him, regardless of his performance. You want him to feel like the best-loved dog, regardless of how he did.

After your score has been recorded, you can get a copy of your score sheet to find out how you and your dog did. If you qualified, you may be in the running for a placement. Wait for the announcement of scores to find out if your dog has placed.

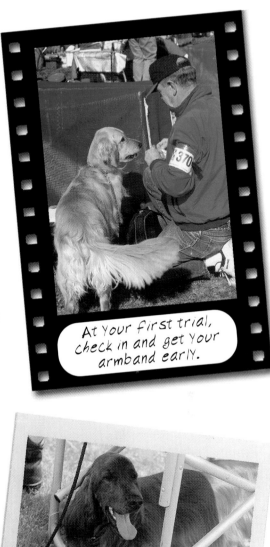

At your first trial, check in and get your armband early.

Whatever the outcome, praise your dog when the trial is over.

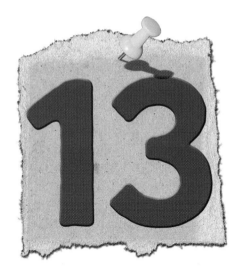

Dog Shows

At dog shows, also called conformation shows, dogs are judged according to the standard approved by the breed club that sanctions the event. Each national club develops a standard for its breed. A standard is a set of qualities that distinguishes one particular breed from another purebred dog. Without standards as a guideline, each breed would not have the characteristics that make it unique. For example, if there was no way to define what a Labrador Retriever looked like, a Lab might look like a Golden Retriever, a Collie, or a mixed breed.

Dog shows are more than just beauty pageants. They enable breeders and fanciers to display breeding stock and determine which dog conforms

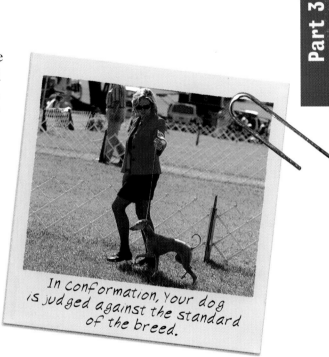

In conformation, your dog is judged against the standard of the breed.

Eligible Breeds

Conformation shows are open to purebred dogs registered with the appropriate breed club. The most popular conformation shows are held by the American Kennel Club (AKC). Entrants must be fully registered with AKC, must be intact (except in Veterans classes), and must be show quality. Show-quality dogs are different from pet-quality dogs in that they do not have cosmetic flaws that would disqualify or severely penalize them.

You can obtain a show-quality dog from a reputable breeder. If you decide that you wish to show dogs, you will first need to become involved in the breed club of your choice because most reputable breeders will sell show-quality prospects only to people that are dedicated to showing and the betterment of the breed.

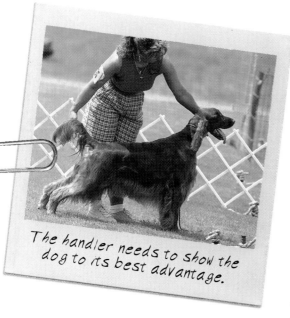

The handler needs to show the dog to its best advantage.

most to the standard. Judges from around the country come to judge dogs based on these standards. Dogs that have not previously become champions vie for points toward a championship. A dog may earn up to five points per show. The amount of points won depends largely on the number of entrants for that specific breed. If the points earned are three or over, the dog is said to have won a *major*. A dog must win two majors under separate judges to qualify for championship. Furthermore, dogs with prior championships may compete for Best of Breed and Best in Show titles along with other competitors.

Does this sound complex? It certainly is! Showing your dog can be time consuming and expensive. But it is fun! For some, showing can become an addiction. People travel all around the country to participate in conformation, and many handlers make a living showing other people's pets. If you have a show-quality purebred dog and this intrigues you, consider showing him.

Training for Conformation

Much of conformation training is about teaching the handler to show the dog properly. In competition, the judge asks the handlers to gait their dogs once around the ring. He then considers each individual dog, examining the face, bite, forelegs, back, and rear legs. On a male, the judge will feel the testicles to confirm that he is intact and has fully descended testicles. Next, the handler will be asked to gait his dog in an up and back, L-shaped, or triangle-shaped pattern. After this examination, the judge will ask the handler to gait the dog to the rear of the line.

Stacking Your Dog

Training for the ring requires that the dog stacks himself or allows himself to be hand stacked. Stacking, standing a dog straight on all fours, accentuates the positive aspects of the dog's conformation and hides flaws that might penalize him. Once stacked, the dog is "baited" with food or treats to produce an attentive expression.

Start training your dog to stack by offering him an interesting tidbit while he is standing. Use the word "stack" and give him a treat when he stands and gives you an alert expression. Dogs are quick at learning this, so wait a few moments before giving the treat. Gradually lengthen the time your dog must hold the stack so that he learns to wait patiently for the treat.

Next, teach your dog to accept having his feet placed in position so that his body is "square" when he stands. After you place one foot and your dog leaves it in the correct position, give him a treat to reinforce that this is what you want him to do. Increase the length of time between your holding the position and giving him the treat. In this way, he will learn how to stand properly and patiently.

Physical Examination

Your dog should be comfortable being touched by other people. Have friends and others examine your dog as a judge would to get him used to the routine. Many professional trainers offer conformation classes that simulate a show ring. You can learn how to properly gait a dog and other useful handling techniques.

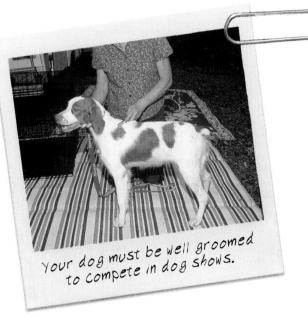

Your dog must be well groomed to compete in dog shows.

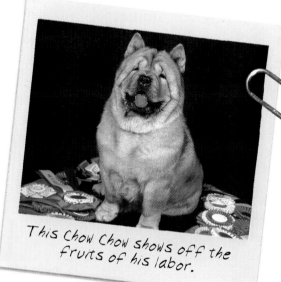

This Chow Chow shows off the fruits of his labor.

Part 3

Looking Good

Last, you must learn how to properly groom your breed for the show ring. Consult with someone who shows your particular breed; he or she can teach you how to properly groom your dog for conformation.

Titles

A dog may place first through fourth in a particular class. If your dog is young and without a title, he may compete in the following classes: 6-9 Months, 9-12 Months, or 12-18 Months. Males compete against males and females compete against females. If your dog is over 18 months, he must be shown in either Novice, American-Bred, Bred-By, or Open Classes.

Novice is for handlers who have never finished a dog. Bred-By can only be entered by breeder/handlers. First-place winners compete for points in the Winners Dog (male) or Winners Bitch (female) class. The winner of this class wins coveted points that go toward a championship. Second place is called Reserved Winners Dog or Reserved Winners Bitch.

The winners of the Winners Dog and Winners Bitch go on to compete against champion dogs for Best of Breed. A dog may also win Best of Winners and Best of Opposite Sex. Dogs that win Best of Breed go on to compete in Best of Group, where winners of each breed in the Group compete against each other. The winner of Group goes on to compete for Best in Show against all the other winners of the Groups.

There are other classes as well, usually only available at specialty shows, which are conformation shows at which only one breed is being judged. These include: Veterans, Working, Brace, Team, and Puppy Classes.

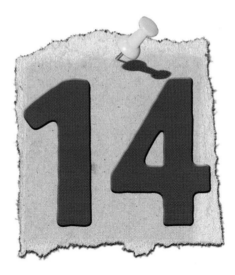

Tracking

Tracking tests require a dog to follow a scent of a particular person and find articles impregnated with the person's scent. AKC tracking allows any purebred dog to compete, although UKC allows mixed breeds as well.

Training the Tracking Dog

Train the tracking dog in increments. Spend no more than 15 minutes a day training your dog so that it is fun, not tedious. You will need a tracking harness; that is, a plain standard walking harness that will not restrict your dog's movement. You will also need a tracking lead, which comes in a variety of sizes. At first, you may use a shorter lead, one less than 20 feet. The required length for AKC tracking leads is between 20 and 40 feet, but while you are training,

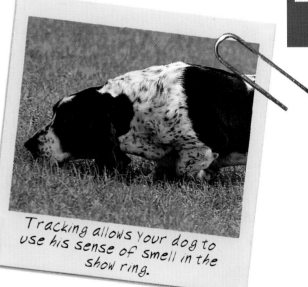

Tracking allows your dog to use his sense of smell in the show ring.

Search and Rescue

Search and rescue differs from competition tracking in a number of ways. Search and rescue dogs (SAR) are trained to find missing humans in a variety of adverse locations and terrain. Unlike tracking, search and rescue often looks for any track, especially in wilderness, disaster, or avalanche conditions. The dogs are trained to find humans, rather than the track and the items, and if the SAR handlers can obtain an item owned by the victim, they use it to show the dog the scent to follow.

There are different types of SAR dogs for different types of adverse conditions. These SAR dogs include:

• Wilderness search dogs

• Avalanche search dogs

• Disaster search dogs

• Urban search dogs

SAR dogs are specialized for each environment and the challenges specific to that environment. The National Association for Search and Rescue (NASAR) certifies search and rescue dogs, but many dogs can be used as SARs through local organizations.

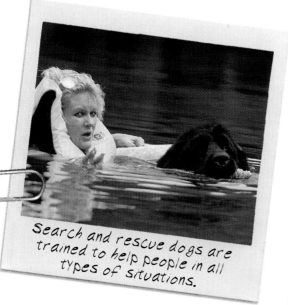

Search and rescue dogs are trained to help people in all types of situations.

you may wish to use a shorter lead for more control and eventually increase your lead size.

You will also need tracking articles. The standard tracking articles are leather gloves and leather wallets. Later on, you will want to teach your dog to locate articles made out of other materials such as cloth, metal, and plastic.

Introducing the Article

Obtain a leather tracking glove or a wallet and use it to tease and play with your dog. Many people will put treats inside the article, so that the article becomes a desirable object for the dog to find. Put your dog in a stay, walk about ten feet away, fill the glove with treats, and put the glove down. Now go back to your dog and say, "Find!" so he will look for the glove. He should be eager to find this "toy." If he's not,

Part 3

lead your dog to the glove and surprise him with the treats and praise. Do this a few times until your dog is excited to find the glove and begins to lead you to it.

You can also lay a trail of treats to the glove to have your dog focus on the ground, rather than the sight of you dropping the glove.

Finding the Article in Different Locations

Next, put the glove in a different location, not far from the first location. Let your dog see you put it down and then return. Tell him, "Find!" Some dogs will go to the first place you left the glove. In this case, encourage your dog to search for the glove, "Find the glove! Find the glove!" Your dog will have to use his nose to sniff out where the glove and goodies are. Some dogs may need some gentle nudging or treats laid along the track, bread-crumb fashion, to help them find the glove in the new spot. Your dog may make a straight line to the glove and the goodies at the first attempt–if he does, that's great. Regardless of whether your dog makes a beeline to the glove or must search for it, continue to try hiding it in different locations until he understands that it may be in any of several different places.

Hiding the Article

Once your dog is comfortable looking for the glove, put him in a place where he cannot see you hide it. Make a short track, drop the glove, and then walk back along that same track. It should be no more than ten feet. Bring him to the start of the track and give the command, "Find!" Your dog may be confused at first. If necessary, help him locate the glove or line the trail

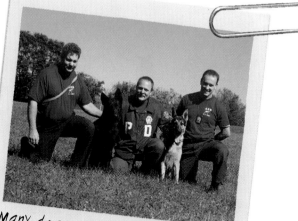

Many dogs work in conjunction with police and fire departments.

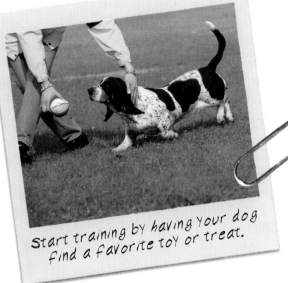

Start training by having your dog find a favorite toy or treat.

Part 3

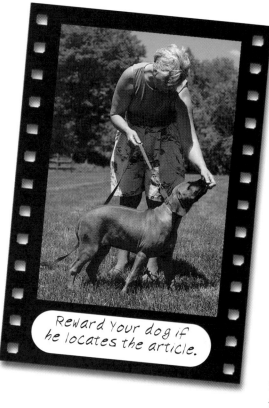

Reward your dog if he locates the article.

Part 3

with treats. When he finds the glove, give him praise and treats. Now, hide the glove while your dog cannot see you doing it and bring him to the track again. Say, "Find!" He may or may not start searching for the glove–again, help him until he starts getting the idea that you want him to find the glove. Use the same established hiding places you used when you first taught your dog to locate the article. He'll remember these and use both his nose and his memory to locate the article.

You may have to lead your dog to the article several times before he gets the idea. You need to stay positive and upbeat in training–you want to encourage your dog to learn, not get frustrated. Always end on a positive note by giving your dog rewards and praise and by playing with him.

Following Someone Else's Track

Once your dog is comfortable following your track and looking for an article, it is time to have your dog follow someone else's track. Use a different glove impregnated with someone else's scent. That person will be the tracklayer for your dog. Start in the same way you did when you introduced your dog to the article, only this time, have the tracklayer show the glove and make the track ten feet away, drop the glove, and return along the same track. Now, your dog must find the glove with the tracklayer's scent. Give the command, "Find!" If your dog is unsure, help lead him to the glove and give him praise and treats. The tracklayer may also give him praise and treats when he finds the glove.

After a few sessions, take your dog away and have the tracklayer lay a short trail and leave the glove with treats. Bring your dog out and give him the command, "Find!" as you had when you hid the article.

Lengthening the Track

As your dog becomes proficient in finding the hidden article, you will want to lengthen the track. Do so a few feet at a time so that your dog becomes used to the distance and starts to rely more on following the track itself. As the distance increases to 15 or more yards, you can make each increase in terms of yards, rather than feet. As you lengthen, keep the track straight until your dog is comfortable going out 20 or more yards to find the article.

Turns in the Track

So far, your track has been in a straight line. Now, have your tracklayer make a definite left or right turn, leave the glove, and return along the same way. You may have to reduce the size of the track by half if it becomes too complicated. Give your dog the command, "Find!" and let him follow the track. If he is using his nose, he will follow the track. Praise him when he follows the track and stop him if he starts to go off-track. When he finally reaches the glove and the treat, give him the treat and praise him, even if he had help. Practice with only one turn for a while.

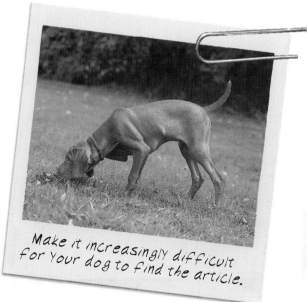

Make it increasingly difficult for your dog to find the article.

Once your dog becomes proficient with one turn in the track, add another. Work with your dog so that he will be certain to pick up the correct track. Again, praise him when he is on the right track and give him assistance when he deviates.

Aging the Track

By now, your dog knows how to follow a track. Now, you must set a track and let it "age" for a certain amount of time. Start with 15 minutes and have your dog follow a simple track. If he successfully tracks the glove, increase the amount of "aging" in 15-minute intervals. You may wish to build up the aging time slowly to be certain that your dog can find the track and complete it successfully.

Multiple Legs

Establish two or more legs, each with a scented article at the end. Start tracking your dog to the first

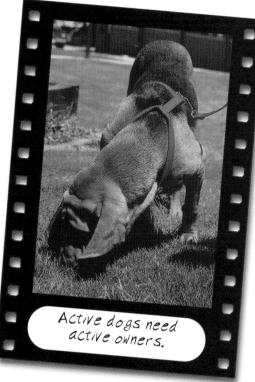

Active dogs need active owners.

Items to Bring to a Tracking Test

Trials are typically held in open fields in parks and at fairgrounds. They may be held at any time of the year. You should consider the weather and location when packing items. Although larger trials held in conjunction with conformation shows and obedience trials may have vendors for food and drink, expect to bring your own. Here is a partial list of items you may want to bring:

√ Water for both you and your dog

√ Water bowls

√ Crate for your dog (exercise pens work well, too)

√ Leash

√ Tracking leash

√ Tracking harness

√ Treats for your dog

√ Plastic mat or ground cover to keep dirt off you and your dog

√ Folding chair

√ Reading material or other entertainment for yourself

√ Toys for your dog

√ Tent or awning

√ Portable fans

√ Raingear or poncho

√ Hat (for sun)

√ Sunglasses and sunblock

√ Cash

article. When he has found it, praise and reward him, and start tracking the next article. Your dog may consider this a new game and may need a little help from you to get started. It shouldn't take long as he will be eager to search for a new article with goodies.

Preparing for the Formal Test

The dog will need a tracking harness and tracking lead. Acceptable tracking lead sizes are between 20 and 40 feet in length. Because there is no time limit on tracking, it's a good idea to bring water for your dog and yourself. You cannot bring food or any other drink.

As you practice for the test, have someone lay a track similar to one that would be used in a real test. This will give you valuable experience. The test has one flag marking the scent and a second flag 30 yards from the first flag, indicating the direction of the track.

Tracking tests may be held in conjunction with conformation shows or obedience trials, but some are held separately. If you do not know where these shows are, contact a local obedience training facility or club or talk to someone who shows their dog in conformation. They should be able to tell you whom to contact regarding local shows, or contact AKC or UKC directly to find out who superintends the shows and trials in your area. Once you obtain the contact information, request the premiums for upcoming trials.

Attending the Trial

Going to your first trial can be daunting, especially if it is held in conjunction with an obedience trial or a conformation show. There are many dogs, loud noises, crowds, and interesting smells. Both you and your dog may find the whole trial distracting. If you can, arrive early so that your dog can become accustomed to the sights and sounds of the event.

AKC Tracking Titles

Tracking Dog (TD): Dogs must pass a certification test in order to enter a tracking test. After qualifying to enter a trial, a dog must pass only one trial for a TD title. A tracking test has the following requirements:

The dog must follow a course or *track* between 440 yards and 500 yards.

The track will have legs of at least 50 yards each.

The track must have three to five turns, two of which turns must be a 90-degree angle. The articles used must be a leather glove or wallet impregnated with the scent of the tracklayer.

The track must be "aged" 30 minutes to 2 hours.

Tracking Dog Excellent (TDX): Certification requirements are the same as for TD. A TDX tracking test requires the following:

The dog must follow a course or *track* between 800 and 1000 yards.

The track will have legs of at least 50 yards long.

The track must have 5 to 7 turns, of which at least 3 turns must be a 90-degree angle.

The four articles used must dissimilar, small personal items of the tracklayer, with the exception of the last item, which may be a glove or wallet.

The track must be "aged" 3 to 5 hours.

Variable Surface Tracking (VST): The dog must earn a VST leg with two judges in agreement to obtain a Variable Surface Tracking (VST) title. A VST tracking test requires the following:

The dog must follow a course or *track* between 600 and 800 yards, with a minimum of three different surfaces, of which two must be devoid of vegetation, concrete, or gravel.

The track will have legs of at least 30 yards long.

The track must have 5 to 7 turns, of which a minimum of 3 turns must be a 90-degree angle.

The four articles used must be dissimilar, small personal items of the tracklayer, including a leather, plastic, metal, and fabric item.

Champion Tracker (CT): The CT title is awarded to dogs that have earned their TD, TDX, and VST titles.

Before the trial, you may receive the judging list and a number as a confirmation in the mail.

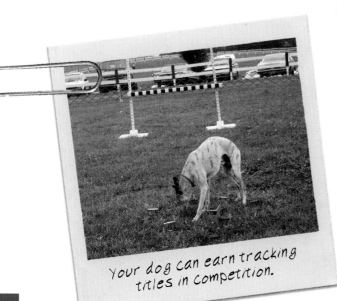

Your dog can earn tracking titles in Competition.

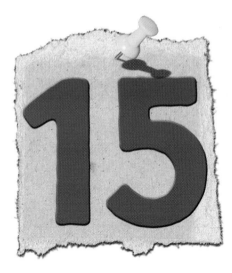

15

Rally-O

Rally-O is not traditional obedience; it's not traditional agility; it's something in between the two, but it stands on its own merits. In Rally classes, which may be either timed or untimed, the team of dog and handler move continuously and perform exercises indicated by a sign at each location. The exercises include, halt, left turn, right turn, about turn, about U-turn, spirals, figure eights, and jumping, as well as basic obedience commands.

After the Judge's "Forward" command, the team is on its own to complete the entire sequence correctly.

Handlers are permitted to talk to or praise their dogs, to clap their hands or pat their legs, or to use

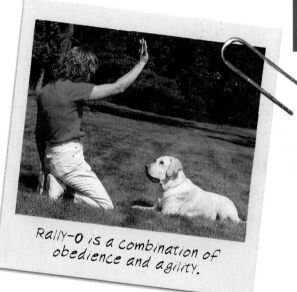

Rally-O is a combination of obedience and agility.

any other verbal means of encouragement. However, they are not permitted to touch their dogs or make corrections with the leash. Each course can have no more than five breaks or stops in the flow of the course of action.

Points are given for each fault in the sequence. Timed courses are judged by taking the run time and adding any fault points to the score. Non-timed course are judged by subtracting any fault points from 200.

Any breed of dog over six months of age, including mixed breeds, can compete in Rally-O. The website of the Association of Pet Dog Trainers (www.apdt.com) has more information on how to get started.

Part Four
Awakening Your Dog's Natural Instincts

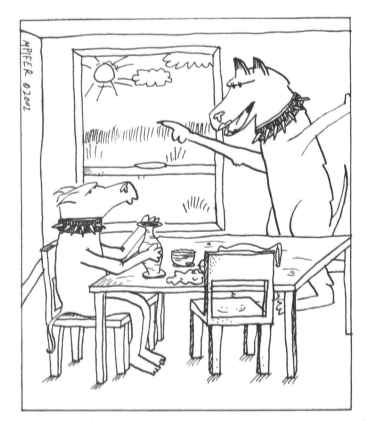

"Pottery! I didn't raise any pup of mine for pottery!
Get outside and guard something!"

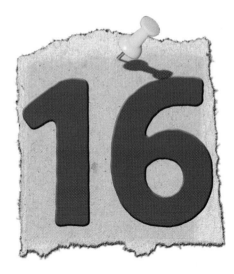

Field Trials

Field trials were developed for owners of certain hunting breeds, i.e., hounds, retrievers, pointers, and spaniels, to prove their dogs' abilities in the field as hunting dogs. Because different dogs were bred for different purposes, there are several types of field trials for each specific breed. For example, in Beagle field trials, the dogs are judged on their accuracy of pursuing rabbits; in pointing breeds, the dogs are judged on finding birds, pointing, and then retrieving downed birds, etc.

Equipment Needed

Training for field trials is an expensive and complex endeavor. Depending on the type of field trial, (such as the Pointing Dog and Retriever Field Trials), you may need to learn how to shoot a rifle along with

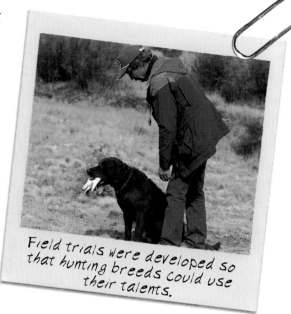

Field trials were developed so that hunting breeds could use their talents.

Eligible Breeds

Field trials are limited to Beagles, Basset Hounds and Dachshunds, pointing breeds, retrievers, and spaniels. Each type of field trial has its own set of rules and requirements as to the performance of the dogs.

Beagles: Beagle field trials are the oldest of the AKC Field Trials. There are three types of Beagle trials, including:

Brace—two or three dogs track rabbits and hares

Small Pack Option (SPO)—packs of seven Beagles each track rabbits and hares

Large Pack Trials—all Beagles at the trial, in one pack, track rabbits and hares

Basset Hounds and Dachshunds: The Basset Hound and Dachshund trials are held separately, but are run in the same format. Basset Hounds or Dachshunds are run in a brace to track small game.

Pointing breeds: Pointing breed field trials are open to Brittany Spaniels, German Shorthaired Pointers, German Wirehaired Pointers, Gordon Setters, Irish Setters, English Setters, Pointers, Vizslas, Weimaraners, and Wirehaired Pointing Griffons. The pointing breeds are run in a brace (pairs) to point birds. After the birds are downed, they must retrieve the downed birds to their owners.

Retrievers: Retriever field trials are open to Chesapeake Bay Retrievers, Curly-Coated Retrievers, Flat-Coated Retrievers, Golden Retrievers, Irish Water Spaniels, and Labrador Retrievers. The retrievers must remember the location of the downed birds, called marking, and must retrieve them.

Spaniels: Spaniel field trials are open to American Cocker Spaniels, English Cocker Spaniels, and English Springer Spaniels. Spaniels must hunt, flush, and retrieve game.

proper firearm safety. Both you and your dog will need appropriate hunter-orange equipment. You will need a whistle, bells, a blank pistol, and other field items.

For Pointing Dog and Retriever field trials, you will need retriever dummies and training scents. You will also need a few dead birds: pheasant, duck, and any other birds required.

Training for Field Trials

Because of the complex nature of field trials, your might want to locate a professional trainer to start your dog off right. Various hunting and game clubs should be able to help you find the right trainer for you and your dog. If you cannot locate a hunting club in your area, contact AKC for a list of nearby organizations. Parent clubs (national organizations) for the respective breeds can be helpful with everything from training to trials.

Teaching Your Dog to Retrieve

If your dog needs to know how to retrieve, you should start by teaching your dog to fetch. Once your dog has learned to fetch, begin using a canvas bumper or plastic dummy designed for training bird dogs.

Toss the dummy ten feet away and send your dog to fetch it. When he returns with the dummy, praise him. If he does not fetch the dummy, walk up with him, put the dummy in his mouth, put him in stay, and walk back. Now call him. If he fails to bring the dummy, work on your fetch command.

Once your dog is comfortable with fetching the dummy, increase the distance. Start at the ten-foot distance and throw the dummy in the same place. Have your dog retrieve it. Now throw the dummy in the same place, turn around, and walk ten feet away from your first position. Now, you have 20 feet between you and the dummy. Tell your dog to fetch. Give him lots of praise when he does it correctly. If he does not, repeat the exercise. Never allow your retriever not to fetch, even if you have to put the dummy in his mouth.

Increase the distance as your dog becomes more proficient in fetching. If at any time your dog has problems with the range, decrease the distance and practice at a shorter distance.

Fetching with a Thrower

At some point, you will not be able to throw the dummy much farther. Instead, have someone throw the dummy for you. The thrower should not throw directly in front of your dog, but rather, off to the left or right so that he does not associate the thrower with the dummy.

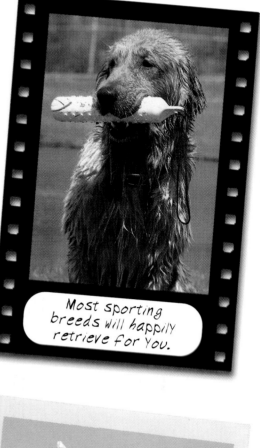

Most sporting breeds will happily retrieve for you.

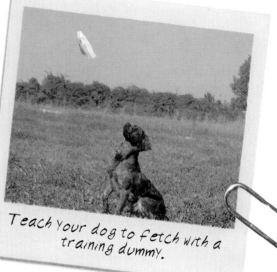

Teach your dog to fetch with a training dummy.

Part 4

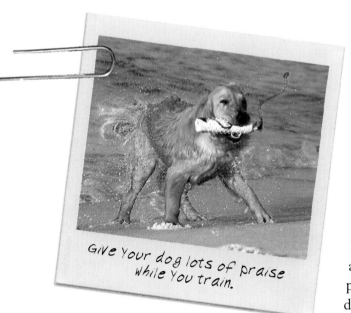

Give your dog lots of praise while you train.

Start at a short distance. Once the dummy is thrown, have your dog retrieve it. Again, you may have to pick up the dummy and put it in your dog's mouth if he doesn't retrieve it.

Retrieving Games

There are various games you can play with your dog to get him to retrieve dummies. One is to lay several dummies in a pattern on the ground, such as a circle, diamond, or square. Lead your dog on leash and as you pass by a dummy, give your dog the retrieve command. Praise him when he picks up the dummy. Take it from him and toss it into a pile inside the circle. Give your dog a command to retrieve another dummy. Repeat the process until all the dummies are in a pile. Then, take a dummy from the pile, throw it, and tell your dog to retrieve it.

These games teach your dog to pick up the dummy when you give the command to retrieve, regardless of whether your dog saw the dummy fall or not.

Training with Birds

Start training with a dead bird. Show your dog the bird and give him the command to retrieve it from your

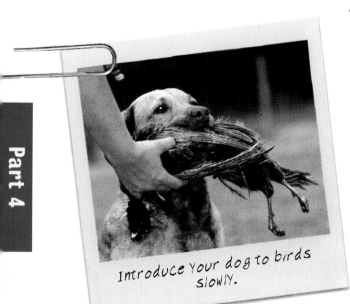

Introduce your dog to birds slowly.

Field Trial Titles
FC—Field Champion
AFC—Amateur Field Champion

Part 4

hands at head height. Praise your dog when he takes the dead bird in his mouth. Now give the command, "Drop it." (You may have to work at removing the dead bird from your dog's mouth, if he isn't proficient at the drop it command.) Praise your dog when he takes the bird on command and again when he releases it.

Now, offer the bird a little lower than mouth level and give the retrieve command. Your dog should have no difficulty in taking the bird from you. Have your dog drop it. Now, continue lowering the bird so that your dog will have to bend his neck to take the bird with each retrieve command. Eventually, you want your dog to pick up the bird from the ground.

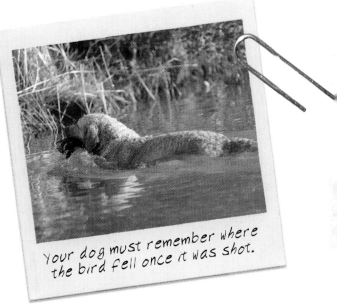

Your dog must remember where the bird fell once it was shot.

Now, increase the range your dog must go to retrieve the bird. Start with just a few feet and then increase the distance as your dog becomes more proficient.

Marking the Shot
Dogs must learn to "mark" the downed bird; meaning that they must remember where the bird fell once it was shot. You can do this with the help of two throwers. Sit your dog some distance away from the two throwers so that they are on your right and left sides. Have the person on your left side throw the dummy. Turn your dog toward it and tell your dog, "Mark!" Now, have the person on the right throw the dummy, a little closer than the left dummy. Turn your dog toward the right dummy and tell your dog, "Mark!" Now, tell your dog to retrieve the right dummy. Once your dog has retrieved the right dummy, have him retrieve the left dummy.

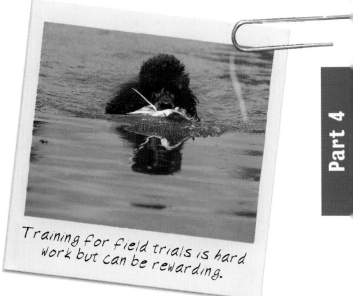

Training for field trials is hard work but can be rewarding.

You may have to lead your dog to the left dummy to have him remember that it is there. Eventually, such training teaches your dog to remember that there is more than one "bird," and he must remember where they all are.

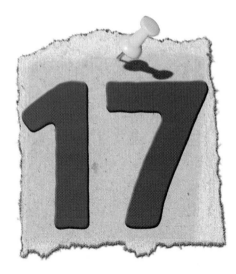

Hunting Tests

Hunting tests prove that a dog is capable of hunting. Unlike field trials, hunting tests are designed so that every dog can be a winner–provided that the dog passes the tests. As in field trials, there are rankings in the hunting tests, but they are less competitive than the field trials.

Equipment Needed

Training for hunting tests is an expensive and complex endeavor (although nowhere near as expensive as field trials!). Depending on the type of hunting test, you may need to learn how to shoot a rifle, as well as proper firearm safety. Both you and your dog will need appropriate hunter-orange apparel. Handler equipment includes a whistle, bells, a blank pistol,

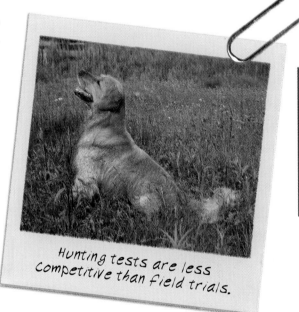

Hunting tests are less competitive than field trials.

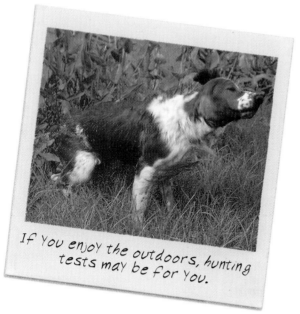

If you enjoy the outdoors, hunting tests may be for you.

Eligible Breeds

A variety of breeds are allowed to compete in hunting tests. These include pointing breeds, flushing spaniels, retrievers, and even Standard Poodles.

Pointing Breeds: Brittany Spaniels, English Setters, German Shorthaired Pointers, German Wirehaired Pointers, Gordon Setters, Irish Setters, Pointers, Vizslas, Weimaraners, and Wirehaired Pointing Griffons

Flushing Spaniels: All spaniels

Retrievers: Chesapeake Bay Retrievers, Curly-Coated Retrievers, Flat-Coated Retrievers, Golden Retrievers, Irish Water Spaniels, and Labrador Retrievers

Standard Poodles

and other field items. Training equipment includes retriever dummies and training scents. You will also need a few dead birds such as pheasant, duck, and any other birds required.

Training

Because of the complex nature of hunting tests, you should locate a professional trainer to start your dog off right. Various hunting clubs should be able to help you find the right trainer for you and your dog. If you cannot locate a hunting club in your area, contact AKC for a list of nearby organizations.

Part 4

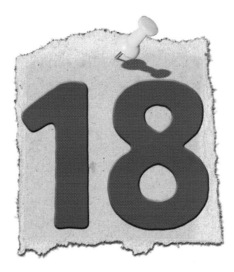

Herding

Herding is one of the dog's oldest professions. Today, dogs are still bred to herd livestock. Dogs and owners compete in herding trials to earn herding titles. Due to different of types livestock and different terrain, humans created a large variety of herding breeds. Some dogs controlled livestock using their eye. Others drove herds from the pasture to the barn at night. Some dogs were bred to protect their herds from animal and human predators.

Equipment Needed

Unless you have your own flock or herd, you will have to "borrow" someone else's stock. These can be sheep, ducks, or cattle. Other than that, you will only need a leash and collar for your dog.

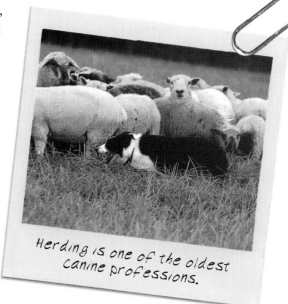

Herding is one of the oldest canine professions.

Eligible Breeds

Herding dogs include dogs from the AKC Herding Group plus Rottweilers and Samoyeds. The AKC recognized Herding Group breeds are: Australian Cattle Dog, Australian Shepherd, Bearded Collie, Belgian Malinois, Belgian Sheepdog, Belgian Tervuren, Border Collie, Bouvier des Flandres, Briard, Canaan Dog, Collie (Rough and Smooth), German Shepherd Dog, Old English Sheepdog, Puli, Shetland Sheepdog, Cardigan Welsh Corgi, and Pembroke Welsh Corgi.

The four major sanctioning organizations for herding are:

The American Kennel Club (AKC)

The Australian Shepherd Club of America (ASCA)

The International Stock Dog Society (ISDS)

The American Herding Breed Association (AHBA)

Training for Herding Tests and Trials

Herding, like other dog sports, has basic commands. These commands tell the dog how to behave when approaching the herd or flock. Although a good herding dog has a natural instinct to work the herd without commands, the best herding dogs have learned specific commands from their shepherds. The actual types of commands may vary. Some handlers use different words, foreign words, or whistles. Dogs that do not have a natural herding instinct can still participate, as much of competition herding depends on the above commands and the handler's capability to command the dog.

The basic herding commands are:

Come to me or go to me–run clockwise around the herd

Away to me–run counterclockwise around the herd

Lie down–stop or lie down

That will do–stop herding

Walk up–go behind the sheep and drive them.

While you might be tempted to teach your dog yourself, it is best to find someone experienced in herding who can help both you and your dog learn together.

You can first teach the dog left ("Away to me") and right ("Go to me"), similar to agility training. Lie down is similar to agility's "Wait" or "Rest," but in order to apply it to herding, you must practice with stock. Your dog should also do a good recall.

Contact AKC, ASCA, or AHBA for information on clubs and trainers in your area. Once you find some prospective trainers, ask if the trainers have experience in training your particular breed. Not all breeds herd the same, and training techniques for one breed may not work with another.

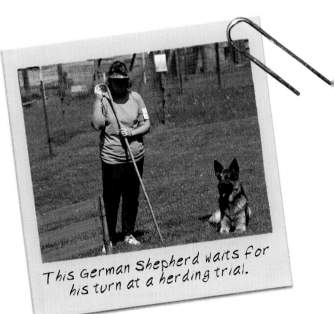

This German Shepherd waits for his turn at a herding trial.

Herding Tests
AKC Herding Test
The AKC Herding Test is designed for novice dogs and handlers to prove the dog's herding ability. The handler has ten minutes for the dog to complete the five basic elements.

Two pylons are placed at each side of the arena along the centerline, within ten feet of the gates. The dog must enter the arena and stop. Next, the dog must move the stock from the first pylon to the second pylon. The dog must then turn the stock at or near the second pylon, and then move the stock

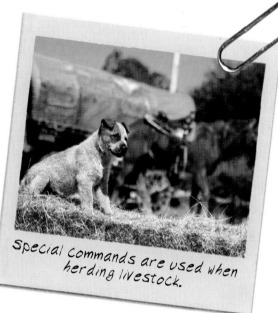

Special commands are used when herding livestock.

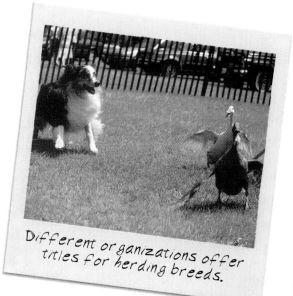

Different organizations offer titles for herding breeds.

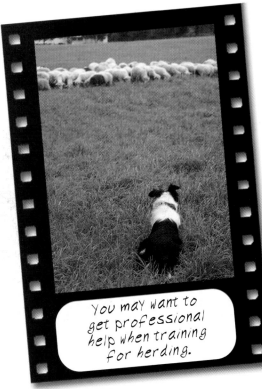

You may want to get professional help when training for herding.

from the second pylon to the first pylon, then turn the stock again toward the second pylon. The handler then issues a stop and recalls the dog.

The AKC Pretrial Test

The AKC Pretrial Test is designed for novice dogs and handlers to demonstrate herding capability just below beginning trial level. The handler has ten minutes for the dog to complete the five basic elements.

There are two gates within the arena. The dog must stop upon entering and then herd the stock through the first gate, through the arena, and then through the second gate. The dog must then turn the stock and move back through the second gate, through the arena, and through the first gate. The dog must then wait while the handler opens the pen. The dog must pen the stock and the handler must close the gate.

The AHBA Herding Capability Tests

The AHBA offers a Herding Capability Test (HCT) title for dogs just starting in herding. The dog must show interest in the livestock by walking around them, gathering them, and moving them toward the handler, driving them toward the handler, or a combination of both.

The dog must show some degree of herding instinct either by nipping, barking, or using his "eye" to control the herd. The dog must show actual instinct, not just chasing or playing with the herd.

The dog must then move the stock around the arena in a controlled fashion and perform a stop and a recall on command.

Part 4

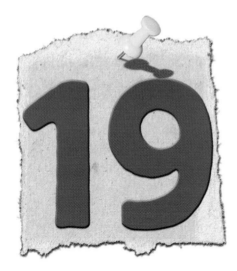

Earthdog Events

Earthdog trials are standardized tests for breeders and owners to measure their dogs' natural working and hunting abilities. Dogs are led to an artificial den where they are encouraged to enter and find the "quarry." The quarry consists of two rats in cages. The dog must show eagerness to pursue the quarry and willingness to "work" the quarry, that is, bark, scratch, and snap at the rats. (The rats are safe within the cage.)

Both AKC and the American Working Terrier Association (AWTA) offer earthdog titles and certifications.

Equipment Needed

The only equipment that the owner of a prospective earthdog needs is a collar and leash. Earthdog tests

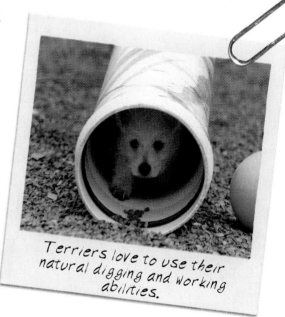

Terriers love to use their natural digging and working abilities.

Earthdog Titles

The AKC offers earthdog titles and an earthdog test. The earthdog test is Introduction to Quarry and is a prerequisite for advanced tests. The titles available for earthdog are: Junior Earthdog (JE), Senior Earthdog (SE), and Master Earthdog (ME).

The American Working Terrier Association offers titles for working terriers. These include both earthdog and hunting. The Working Certificate (WC) title, Hunting Certificate (HC) title, and Certificate of Gameness (CG) are open to all breeds, not just terriers.

Eligible Breeds

Breeds eligible to participate in AKC Earthdog Trials are Dachshunds, Australian Terriers, Bedlington Terriers, Border Terriers, Cairn Terriers, Dandie Dinmont Terriers, Fox Terriers (Smooth and Wirehaired), Jack Russell Terriers, Lakeland Terriers, Manchester Terriers, Miniature Bull Terriers, Miniature Schnauzers, Norfolk Terriers, Norwich Terriers, Scottish Terriers, Sealyham Terriers, Silky Terriers, Skye Terriers, Welsh Terriers, and West Highland White Terriers.

In addition to these breeds, the American Working Terrier Association recognizes Patterdale Terriers and Jadgterriers. Any breed can earn a Working Certificate (WC) and Hunting Certificate (HC) with AWTA.

and practices are generally held by local terrier and Dachshund clubs. Since the "den" requires significant earthwork, i.e., digging, elaborate supports, and quarry, the cost of setting up an earthdog test in your own backyard is usually cost-prohibitive.

Training

Locate a local club that sponsors earthdog tests, trials, and training. Contact a local training facility or terrier or Dachshund breed club for information regarding local earthdog training in your area. If you cannot locate a club that sponsors earthdog events, contact the AKC or AWTA directly for a listing of nearby earthdog clubs.

Many clubs hold practice sessions or practice runs after trials. Introduce your dog into the "den" by offering encouragement. Most young terriers will catch the scent of the quarry and start down the tunnel. A few may need encouragement. You may need a toy or food to entice your dog to enter the den. Some dogs need to be shown the rats and get a good sniff before venturing into the tunnel after them. It is important to mention here that all quarry is caged and protected from contact with the dogs in all AKC earthdog work

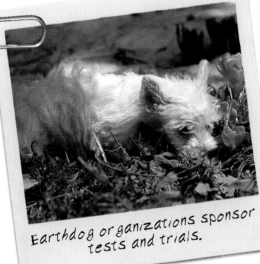

Earthdog organizations sponsor tests and trials.

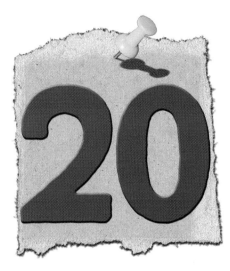

Lure Coursing

Lure coursing is a sport that allows sighthound owners to prove their dogs' coursing instinct. The sighthound was originally bred for spotting prey from great distances and pursuing it. The most common sighthound, the racing Greyhound, still displays these instincts when running on a racetrack. However, for those owners who do not wish to race competitively, lure coursing offers the excitement and challenge of coursing prey without the actual hunt.

The "lure" is a paper bag or a piece of rabbit skin tied to a string attached to the lure machine. The lure is drawn through a course made up of pulleys in a field a minimum of five acres in size. When released, the lure travels at about 40 miles per hour through the

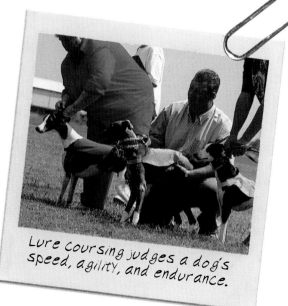

Lure coursing judges a dog's speed, agility, and endurance.

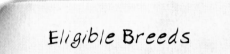

Eligible Breeds

In both AKC and ASFA, breeds eligible to compete include: Afghan Hounds, Basenjis, Borzois, Greyhounds, Ibizan Hounds, Irish Wolfhounds, Italian Greyhounds, Pharaoh Hounds, Rhodesian Ridgebacks, Salukis, Scottish Deerhounds, and Whippets. Mixed breeds and other purebreds may not compete for titles. However, most sighthound clubs offer practice run-throughs that anyone may participate in for a fee.

field in front of the chasing dogs.

Both AKC and American Sighthound Field Association (ASFA) sanction lure coursing. The dog is judged on speed, agility, ability to follow the lure, overall ability, and endurance.

Equipment Needed

Lure coursing equipment is large and costly. The complex series of cables and the lure-coursing machine can be cost-prohibitive to most people. Setting up a lure course is generally impractical because it requires a fair amount of acreage, a motor, and pulleys. Most sighthound owners train with a club or use a bag on a string as a lure. Many offer practice time after competitions to anyone willing to pay a few dollars to run a lure course. Take advantage of any opportunity to train if a club in your area offers lure coursing practice or matches. Contact local clubs to find out when their next practice is scheduled.

You may wish to use a Greyhound muzzle during the dog's run. Sighthounds often get excited and may bite at the pulleys, risking broken teeth. Lure coursing can cause injuries, especially if the dog catches a leg on the string while the lure is running.

Training

Take a white plastic bag and tie it to a long string. This will be your lure. If you have an enclosed area, you will want to let your dog off leash and start dragging the lure. You may have to pull it in short, jerky movements to entice your dog at first. Your dog should chase after the bag. Give him plenty of praise when he shows interest.

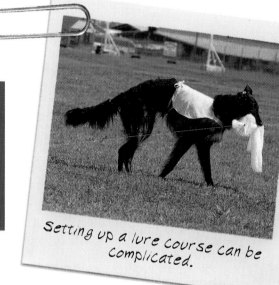

Setting up a lure course can be complicated.

Lure Coursing Titles

The following titles are available in AKC events:

Junior Courser (JC)—Dog must receive two certifications from two different judges on two different courses.

Senior Courser (SC)—Dog must have a Junior Courser title and must qualify in four Open Stakes courses under two different judges. The dog must run with another dog to qualify.

Master Courser (MC)—Dog must have a Senior Courser title and have earned 25 qualifying scores in Open Stakes, Open Veterans, or Specials Stakes.

Field Champion (FC)—Dog must earn 15 championship points, including 2 first placements of 3 points or more. One point must be earned against a hound of the same breed. Points depend on breed and number of dogs in the competition.

Lure Courser Excellent (LCX)—Dog must have a Field Champion title and 45 championship points. This is a cumulative title and dogs are able to advance to LCX II, LCX III, etc. for each 45 championship points accrued.

The ASFA offers these titles:

Field Champion (FCh.)—Dog must earn 100 points in Open Stakes and have 2 first place finishes or 1 first place and 2 second place finishes.

Lure Courser of Merit (LCM)—Dog must earn 300 points in Field Champion Stakes and have 4 first place finishes.

Lure coursing is not for dog-aggressive dogs. Although your dog earns his Junior Courser title without running with another dog, later titles require that two or more dogs run together. Your dog should be more interested in chasing the lure than in playing or fighting with other dogs. Dogs that interfere with other dogs can be dismissed or disqualified.

Lure coursing is mostly instinctual. Sighthounds will chase after movement, which is why you should never allow your sighthound to run loose. A paper blowing in the wind or a rabbit can divert your sighthound for miles.

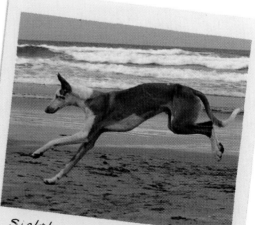

Sighthounds have the inherent instinct to chase after prey.

Part 4

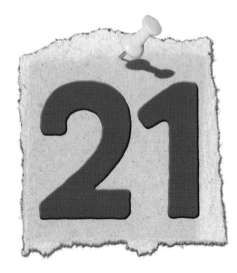

21

Schutzhund

The word "schutzhund" means "protection dog" in German. Although protection is a part of Schutzhund training, it comprises only a third of the actual tests. Dogs are tested in obedience, tracking, and protection. Schutzhund was originally developed for German Shepherd Dogs in Germany to measure their working ability.

There are two major Schutzhund organizations within the United States: United Schutzhund Clubs of America and DVG America.

What Schutzhund is *Not*

Schutzhund is not "attack dog" or "guard dog" training, although it does teach a dog to attack *on command*. It does *not* intend to make the dog a

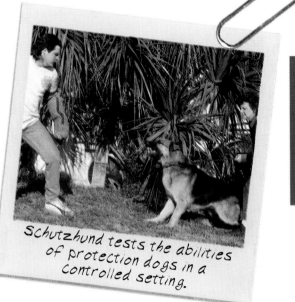

Schutzhund tests the abilities of protection dogs in a controlled setting.

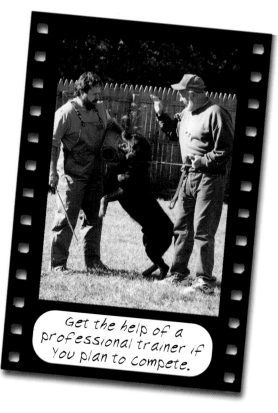

Get the help of a professional trainer if you plan to compete.

"loaded weapon," nor does it make a dog aggressive. While protection training is indeed a part of Schutzhund, the dog is well-disciplined and, therefore, only exhibits those behaviors when there is danger to the handler (an attacking adversary) or in response to a command. Dangerous, unreliable dogs will have a difficult, if not impossible, time passing Schutzhund's rigorous requirements.

Eligible Breeds

Any dog may compete in Schutzhund trials, although there is a natural size limitation because of hurdles and A-frames (for example, the dog must jump a 40-inch hurdle and climb a 6-foot A-frame).

Titles

Begleithund (Bh)

The Begleithund title (Bh) means "companion dog." Unlike the Companion Dog title in AKC, the Bh title requires traffic exercises, that is, the dog must perform when pedestrian traffic is present.

Schutzhund I (SchH1), Schutzhund II (SchH2), Schutzhund III (SchH3)

These Schutzhund titles requires that a dog be tested in obedience, tracking, and protection.

Schutzhund A (SchHA)

The examination for the Schutzhund A (SchHA) title is the same as the SchH1 examination, except that the tracking portion of the test is excluded.

FH1 and FH2

These are advanced tracking titles for dogs and handlers wishing to work further on tracking beyond a SchH3 title.

Watch Dog Test (WH)

The examination for the Watch Dog (WH) title tests for basic watchdog instinct. The watchdog test is open to all breeds.

Part 4

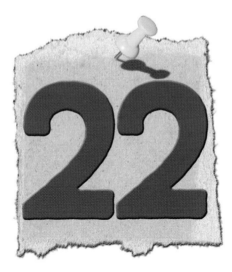

Carting

Is your dog a giant breed? Is he capable of pulling a wagon while still being calm and collected? If so, your dog might be perfect for carting.

While there are many similarities to sledding rigs and carts, traditional carting comes from Northern Europe where draft breeds originated. These dogs generally pulled a small cart, travois, or wagon. Unlike sledding rigs or carts, the wagons only needed one dog to pull.

Equipment Needed

Your dog will need a harness. Depending on the type of vehicle, the harness can be a parade harness, a siwash harness, or a draft harness. The parade harness is common. It has a padded strap across the

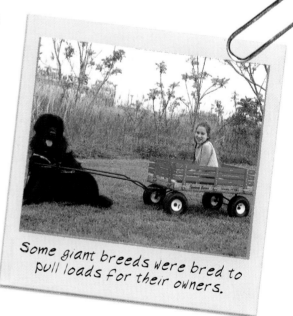

Some giant breeds were bred to pull loads for their owners.

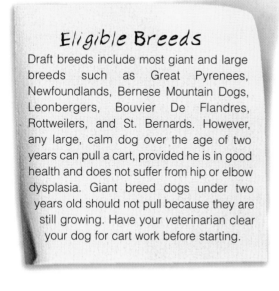

Eligible Breeds

Draft breeds include most giant and large breeds such as Great Pyrenees, Newfoundlands, Bernese Mountain Dogs, Leonbergers, Bouvier De Flandres, Rottweilers, and St. Bernards. However, any large, calm dog over the age of two years can pull a cart, provided he is in good health and does not suffer from hip or elbow dysplasia. Giant breed dogs under two years old should not pull because they are still growing. Have your veterinarian clear your dog for cart work before starting.

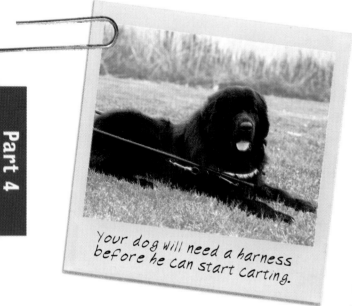

Your dog will need a harness before he can start carting.

chest and back and attaches to either poles or straps. The siwash harness is similar to the weightpull harness, but does not have the spreader bar or singletree. The draft harness looks like a miniature version of a horse draft harness.

The vehicle can be a wagon, cart, or travois. The wagon is perhaps the best vehicle because it has four wheels and does not put weight on the dog's back like the cart and travois. The cart has two wheels and places some of the burden on the dog's back; therefore, you should never have a heavy load in it. The travois is a drag vehicle and best for transporting over rough terrain, but again, because the dog's back must support some of the weight, it is very important to keep the loads light.

Teaching Your Dog to Pull a Cart

Not surprisingly, many of the commands used in carting are the same ones that are used in sledding. "Hike," "Whoa," "Gee," and "Haw" are all used to command the carting dog. Start by teaching your dog to become accustomed to the harness. Put the harness on and give your dog treats every time he wears it.

Teach your dog to pull and learn commands. Begin drag training and start by hooking up a small piece of firewood to your dog's harness to serve as a drag. Your dog will become accustomed dragging this noisy, bouncy thing behind him.

Once your dog is confident with the commands and used to the drag, you can introduce the wagon or cart.

Part 4

Let him sniff and inspect the cart or wagon before getting in harness. If you have successfully drag-trained the dog, the wagon should not be a cause for concern. You may need to use food as a lure and give plenty of praise and treats. Choose a place with level ground that does not have too many distractions. Say, "Hike" and see if your dog is willing to pull. If your dog is nervous about pulling, try snapping on a leash and gently coax him. Offer him treats to lure him forward and give him treats and praise with each step.

These first training sessions should be no more than ten minutes long each day. Afterward, unhitch the wagon, remove the harness, and play with you dog. This will be his reward for doing such a good job. Once your dog becomes more accustomed to the cart or wagon, slowly increase the amount of time in harness. After your dog becomes used to pulling the cart, you can start adding weight slowly.

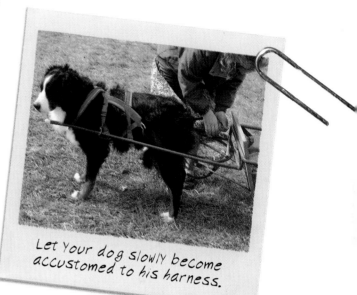

Let your dog slowly become accustomed to his harness.

Where to Go from Here

National breed clubs (parent clubs) offer titles and drafting competitions. Contact the Bernese Mountain Dog Club of America, Saint Bernard Club of America, North American Working Bouvier Association, Newfoundland Club of America, or the American Rottweiler Club for more information concerning breed club titles. (Contact information can be found in the Resource section of this book.)

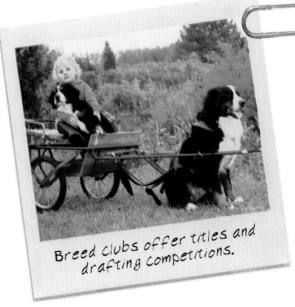

Breed clubs offer titles and drafting competitions.

Part 4

Draft Dog Titles

Bernese Mountain Dog Club of America:

Novice Draft Dog (NDD), Draft Dog (DD), Brace Novice Draft Dog, (BNDD), Brace Draft Dog (BDD)

Newfoundland Club of America:

Draft Dog (DD), Team Draft Dog (TDD)

St. Bernard Club of America:

Draft Dog (DD), Team Draft Dog (TDD)

American Rottweiler Club:

Carting Started (CS), Carting Intermediate (CI), Carting Excellent (CE)

Part 4

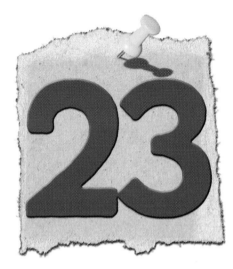

23

Weightpulling

Weightpulling is a competition where a dog in harness pulls a sled or a cart with heavy weights a distance of 16 feet. Any healthy dog is capable of weightpulling. Most dogs, even small dogs, are capable of pulling many times their weight, provided they are properly trained and are physically sound. Dogs enjoy the work and competition as much, if not more so, as their owners do. Dogs pull for the sheer enjoyment and are not coerced in any fashion.

If weightpulling appeals to you, be aware that your dog must be older than 1 year and younger than 12 years in order to compete. Other weightpulling sanctioning bodies may have different age requirements. In large breeds, such as Alaskan

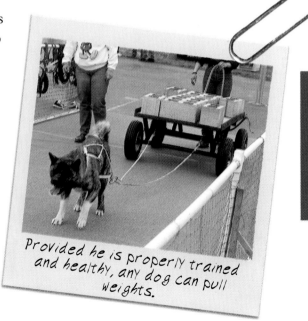

Provided he is properly trained and healthy, any dog can pull weights.

Eligible Breeds

In competition, weightpulls are not limited to Northern breeds, nor are they limited to a specific size. There are 6 weight classes in the International Weight Pull Association's (IWPA) sanctioned pulls, which includes dogs under 35 pounds, dogs between 35 and 60 pounds, dogs between 60 and 80 pounds, dogs between 80 and 100 pounds, dogs between 100 and 120 pounds, and dogs over 120 pounds. Other sanctioning bodies may have different weight classes and different rules.

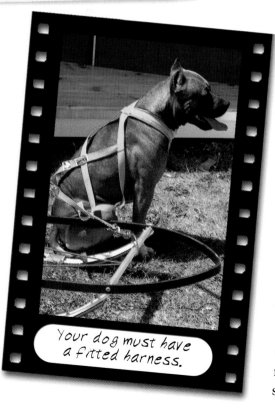

Your dog must have a fitted harness.

Malamutes and Newfoundlands, owners may wish to wait until their dogs are at least 18 months of age. If you have a young dog, ask your veterinarian when your dog will be able to participate in weightpulls and weightpull training.

Equipment Needed

Weightpulling requires very little equipment, which makes it an inexpensive sport. The dog must have a properly-fitted weightpull harness. Most owners start training their dogs using a small tire hooked to a long chain behind the harness's tug ring. If you wish to start out with a lighter weight, screw a large eyebolt into the top of a fence post, a 2 x 4 plank, or a stick of firewood. You can then attach a rope or an old leash to the drag.

Do *not* use mushing harnesses or so-called "roading" harnesses (sometimes available at pet stores). These can cause severe injury to a dog when used in freighting and weightpulling. The correct harness is the siwash freighting harness that you can purchase from weightpulling and mushing outfitters. This harness is heavily padded with foam or synthetic sheepskin. It is similar to the mushing X-back harness, as it crisscrosses across the back. However, unlike mushing harnesses, the harness straps do not meet at the base of the tail on top of the rump. Instead, they run the length of the dog, just below the elbow, and meet behind the dog's flank to a ring. Just behind the flank is a spreader bar or "singletree"–a round or square half-inch dowel that holds the straps apart, enabling the dog to "dig in" with his hind legs. Do not weightpull with a harness that does not have a spreader bar.

Teaching Your Dog to Weightpull

Once your dog is comfortable with basic drag training, you can start with the piece of firewood or 2 x 4 with an eyebolt. Hook one end of a rope or chain to the tug ring and the other end to the eyebolt. Choose a level area covered in dirt. Snap a leash on your dog's collar and lead him forward in a straight line. He should feel the weight of the drag. If the weight is not too heavy or if your dog is a determined puller, he may charge through without giving the weight a second thought. Use a treat to lure his head lower as he pulls so that he learns the correct form. You want his head low so that he can use his shoulders and chest to pull the weight. Praise him and give him the treat.

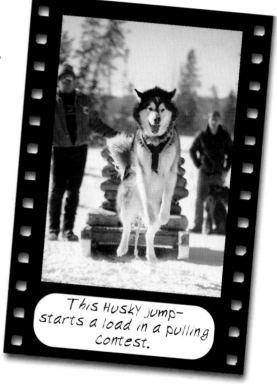

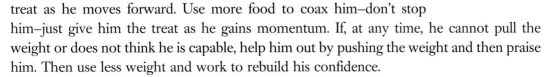

This Husky jump-starts a load in a pulling contest.

If your dog hesitates, use food to lure him forward. Keep it low and just a few inches out of his reach. If the weight is not too much, he should make an attempt to get the treat. Praise him and give him the treat as he moves forward. Use more food to coax him–don't stop him–just give him the treat as he gains momentum. If, at any time, he cannot pull the weight or does not think he is capable, help him out by pushing the weight and then praise him. Then use less weight and work to rebuild his confidence.

Weightpulling is mostly a mental exercise for the dog. While good condition is of prime importance, your dog must be convinced he can pull the weight. Once your dog shows confidence, you should practice with that same weight for 10 starts at about 30 feet. After each pull or each two to three pulls, unhook the weight and walk your dog around to stretch out his muscles. With each pull, use a command to pull, such as "Hike!" or "Dig!" Train for two weeks once or twice a day. After two weeks, your dog should become comfortable with the drag.

The next step is to switch to a fence post with an eyebolt. At this phase, decide whether you wish to call your dog from the front or "drive" him from behind. Both have their

Part 4

Depending on his size, gradually build up the weight your dog pulls.

Competitive weight pulls are fun for both dog and owner.

advantages. Many dogs love coming to their owners; thus, the reward is heartfelt hugs and kisses. Still, some dogs love having their owners drive them from behind, feeling that this is more a team effort. Try both—no doubt one will seem more natural to you. You will also want to teach your dog the stay command, if he does not know already. Put him on a long leash, such as a tracking leash, give him the stay command, and have someone hold him while you take your position, either to call him or drive him. Give him a moment or two to wait, and then command him to pull. Again, give him two weeks of training with the new drag.

Assuming your dog is not a toy breed or small breed, the next step is to use a small tire from a compact passenger car as a drag. Lay the tire on its side so it is flat on the ground. Use chains to hook the tire to your dog's tug. Again, practice good form: head lowered, shoulders forward. As your dog becomes used to the weight, start adding to it. Chains or bricks added slowly will increase the drag. You will first start with the car tire only. Have your dog pull the weight for 5 to 10 starts a distance of 30 feet. Then, increase the weight and practice for 5 to 10 starts at 25 feet. Increase the weight again and have your dog pull the weight 20 feet for 2 to 5 starts. The last increase in weight should be close to your dog's maximum, and he should only pull one to three times. Then, remove some weight and have your dog pull the lower weight. The workout should consist of 20 to 35 starts with rests and walks between each start.

If at any time your dog balks at the weight, help him with it so he can finish the pull. Reduce the weight and have him pull it. End on a positive note. Practice every day or every other day, but do not try to go for too much too soon.

Competitive Weightpulling

Weightpull competitions are fun and exciting for both dogs and owners. The competition requires that the dogs weigh in to determine their classes. You cannot use a leash, food, toys, or anything that might be considered a motivator while the dog is weightpulling. The dog must pull the assigned weight 16 feet within 1 minute, or as determined by the sponsoring organization's rules.

Part 4

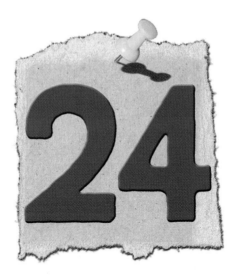

Skijoring

Skijoring is a sport where the dog pulls his owner on skis. Most dogs that are healthy and over 30 pounds can be skijoring dogs. A skijoring dog need not be a Northern breed, but certainly the drive to pull and the thick double coat has its advantages. You should have your veterinarian check your dog's hips and elbows for dysplasia before starting to skijor. If your dog is still a puppy, you can begin harness and light drag training, but you should not have him pull you until he is at least one year old. Before your dog does any pulling, ask your veterinarian for a clean bill of health.

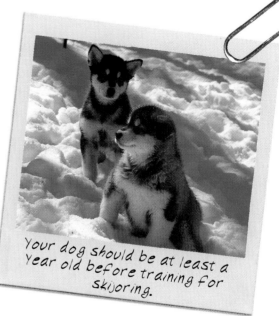

Your dog should be at least a year old before training for skijoring.

Your Ability as a Skier

You don't need to be an expert skier to try skijoring, but knowing how to stop, skate, and pole are all

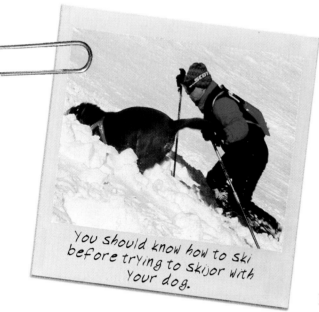

You should know how to ski before trying to skijor with your dog.

Eligible Breeds

Any breed of dog can compete in skijoring.

If your dog is healthy and over 30 pounds, he can skijor.

useful things to know. One should also know how to fall correctly to avoid injury. If this is your first time on skis or if you are not a good skier, consider taking skiing lessons to learn the rudiments of the sport.

You will need to be able to help your dog pull you, especially if you are planning to compete. Learning to skate and pole smoothly without disrupting your dog's rhythm is very important, especially if you are planning to enter skijoring competitions.

Equipment

• Ski equipment and clothing. The type of skis is strictly up to you, but many people prefer cross-country skis because they allow the owner to work behind the dog more easily. However, this is strictly based on your preference and overall ability.

• Skijoring belt or harness. This type of belt or harness can be made from leather or nylon. It should be padded for your comfort and have a quick-release snap in case you must quickly free yourself from your dog.

• Towline and shock cord. The towline is made from spliced polyethylene rope that attaches one, two, or three dogs to the skijorer. It should be long enough to provide a safe buffer zone for your dog in case you lose control. The shock cord, constructed from bungee, attaches to the towline and protects the dog from hard jolts.

Part 4

• X-back or H-back racing harness. These are the same harnesses used by mushers.

• Booties to protect your dog's paws from snowballing and abrasive snow.

• A dog coat for extremely cold weather or if your dog has a short coat.

Teaching Your Dog to Skijor

Always start out with one dog. Train your dog to pull. Once you feel comfortable with your dog's training, you can try skijoring. Do not do this alone! Have a friend who is a proficient skier or who can follow you down a trail come with you. Choose an uncrowded, flat, wide trail or area for your first run. Start by putting your dog in a stay and have your friend hold him while you hook him up to your skijoring belt. Use the commands "Hike" to go and "Whoa" to stop, just as you had in pull training.

Your first few runs should be short as you begin to learn how to help your dog tow you. You will have to worry about stopping correctly to avoid hitting your dog and making a smooth transition going forward. As your confidence builds, you can start working toward skijoring for a mile or more. Once you feel confident with your dog's abilities–and your abilities as well–you can add a second skijor dog. Just be certain that the second dog is as well trained as your first and that both get along. You don't need to break up a dogfight in the middle of a trail!

Where to Go from Here

Most skijoring competitions are sprint races between three to five miles, although there are skijoring distance races. These distance races may go 20 miles or more. Skijor races are divided into classes: 1-, 2-, or 3-dog skijor. These races are usually run over a weekend with two heats. The combined time of both heats make up your final time for the race. The International Sled Dog Racing Association (ISDRA) sanctions skijor races.

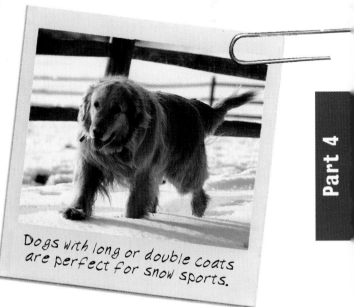

Dogs with long or double coats are perfect for snow sports.

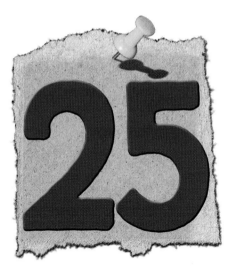

Sledding

Do the words "sled dogs" and "mushing" conjure romantic images of a dog team traveling across the wilds of the frozen north? If you desire the thrill of riding behind your own team of Huskies or Malamutes, know that you're in good company. In this modern age, sled dog racing is a popular sport, not only in Alaska, but in the lower 48 as well.

Unlike Jack London's world of the arctic, modern-day sled dogs receive excellent care. Dog food manufacturers and veterinary schools have made the sled dog's diet and performance the subject of extensive research. Race organizations ban the use of steroids and medications that seek to enhance performance or mask symptoms of a serious

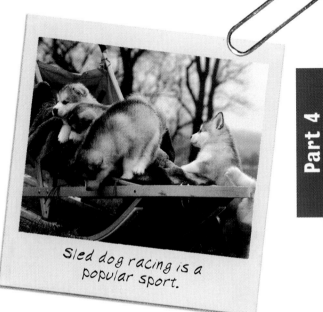

Sled dog racing is a popular sport.

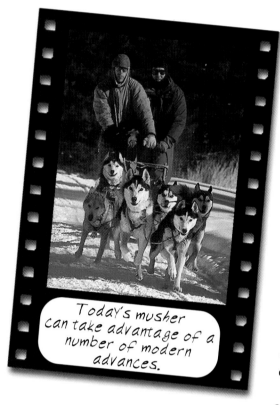

Today's musher can take advantage of a number of modern advances.

condition. Likewise, these organizations prohibit abusive treatment of sled dogs at any race. Major sanctioning bodies such as the International Sled Dog Racing Association (ISDRA) ban whips. In any race, the welfare of the dogs is paramount.

The modern musher has a baffling number of advances at his or her disposal. Sleds made from aluminum or composite materials are readily available if the musher seeks an "edge" over the competition. Sports drinks for sled dogs ensure glycogen repletion. Gore-Tex and other synthetic fibers assure keeping the musher dry as well as warm.

Women and men compete equally in these races, as the 1980s saw with Iditarod winners Libby Riddles and Susan Butcher. In this sport, there are as many women competing as there are men. Several race organizations are offering youth races as well to encourage competition and good sportsmanship.

Mushing, however, is an expensive sport. Many beginners, not understanding the overall cost in time and money, quickly collect dogs only to discover the expense and hassle involved. These people leave the sport almost as quickly as they come in–often at the dogs' expense. Organizations such as Mush with PRIDE educate novice mushers on their responsibilities as sled dog owners.

If you are interested in mushing, try skijoring first to see if you enjoy driving dogs. If you are still interested in mushing, consider running a three-dog team. Most municipalities allow only two or three dogs per household, so a three-dog team is usually what most novice mushers race. After that, you will have a major decision to make: whether to move to an area that will allow multiple dogs or to be satisfied with running a three-dog team. No matter where you move, be certain that you understand the zoning ordinances and covenants. Otherwise, you will have problems with the local code enforcement officer and animal control. You cannot hide 10 or 20 dogs from your neighbors or animal control for very long!

Eligible Breeds

If your dog is healthy and over 30 pounds, he can be a sled dog. A sled dog need not be a Northern breed—many successful teams have run with nonstandard dogs such as German Shorthaired Pointers and Coonhounds. Before you start mushing, you should have your veterinarian check your dog's hips and elbows for dysplasia. If you have a puppy, you can began harness and light drag training, but you should not race him until at least a year. Always have your veterinarian give him a clean bill of health before beginning sled dog training.

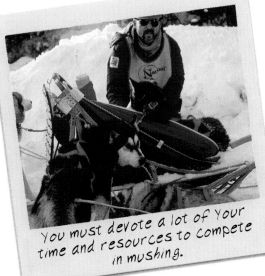

You must devote a lot of your time and resources to compete in mushing.

The problem of multiple dogs goes beyond zoning. You must properly feed, house, exercise, and clean up after your dogs. You cannot take a break from them. Mushing is more of a lifestyle than a sport.

How Many Dogs do you Need?

How many dogs make a team? One dog can pull a person and sled over flat terrain, but in order to race, you must have a minimum of three dogs for a competitive dog team. Sprint races allow an unlimited number of dogs per team. Distance races usually allow 6, 10, 12, or 16 dogs in a team, depending on the race.

Snow or No Snow

Surprisingly, many mushers train in areas where snow is scarce during part or all of the training season. To compensate for lack of snow, mushers train using specially designed carts or rigs. Unlike those used in carting, these rigs are somewhat chariot-like. They are three- or four-wheeled vehicles that the musher stands in and steers while the dogs pull them. They can be very unstable and prone to tipping over if the musher uses a large, powerful team.

Part 4

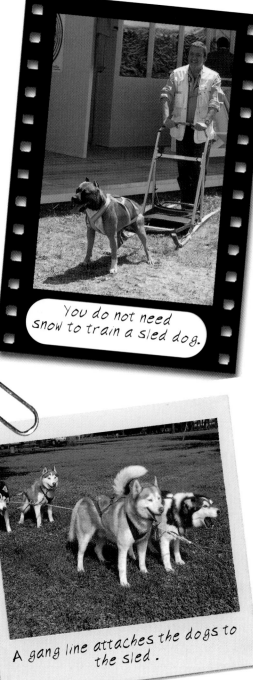

You do not need snow to train a sled dog.

A gang line attaches the dogs to the sled.

Many mushers now use ATVs or all terrain vehicles for training sled teams on dirt. ATVs offer more control than carts with excellent braking and power to help teams on hills. If you choose to train with an ATV, be certain to purchase a four-wheel model. Three-wheel models are less stable and more prone to accidents.

Types of Racing

There are several different types of racing:

Long distance racing–made famous by such races as the Iditarod–is a course usually above 250 miles long and requires over 12 dogs.

Sprint racing, a popular form of sled dog racing, is a course anywhere from 3 to 30 miles long. Limited class sprint racing is measured as one mile per dog. Therefore, a three-dog race will average three miles. There are also 4, 6, 8, and 10 dog races in the Limited class. Unlimited class races tend to be 20 to 30 miles long. There are usually two heats in a sprint race, run on consecutive days.

Mid-distance races are anywhere from 20 to 250 miles and usually require 6, 10, or more dogs.

Stage races, a new type of racing, are run for a set number of miles each day for two to ten days. Stage races are a hybrid compromise between sprint racing and distance racing. The number of dogs depends on the race. As stage racing is relatively new, the rules are evolving.

Cart racing is done with wheeled carts, rigs, or gigs on dirt. Like sprint races, cart races are usually run one mile per dog. Some organizations are offering distance cart races, where the mileage may be 15 to 25 miles per heat.

Part 4

Freight racing is a type of race where a team must pull a certain amount of weight per dog over a few miles. This type of racing is not as popular as other types.

Equipment

Sled–either a basket sled or a toboggan sled (Basket sleds are more often used for shorter races on groomed trails because they are lighter. Toboggans are used for distance races where there is the need to carry supplies over ungroomed trails.)

Gang line–the line that attaches the dogs to the sled

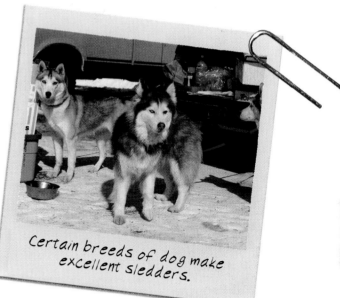

Certain breeds of dog make excellent sledders.

X-back or H-back harnesses–one per dog

Sled bag–to carry equipment or an injured dog

Snow hook–to anchor the sled when stopped

Snub lines–an alternative method to tying off the sled

Shock cord–a thick bungee that protects the dogs from hard jolts

Booties–to protect the dogs' feet from abrasive snow and to prevent snowballing

Dog coats–to provide extra warmth in extreme conditions

Training for Sledding

Once you have determined that you want a sled team, the next step is to determine whether you will be running for competition or for fun. If you choose competition, the top teams are almost all Alaskan Huskies. Some Siberian Husky teams, mostly out of Leonhard Seppala and Seppala-derived racing lines, are very competitive with Alaskan Husky teams. The current trend in Alaskan Huskies is to cross in German Shorthaired Pointers for speed–top North American teams run Alaskan/ Shorthair crosses.

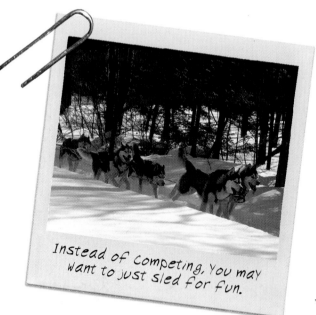

Instead of competing, you may want to just sled for fun.

If you choose to run competitively with your own breed, many clubs offer purebred or Siberian Husky awards. The team must consist of all the same breed, such as all Siberian Husky, all Samoyed, or all Alaskan Malamute. Alaskan Huskies are not considered a purebred dog and therefore cannot compete for purebred awards. Many breed clubs offer their own working titles for sledding. Contact your dog's national breed club for more information.

If you choose to sled for fun, you can decide what type of team to run, where you want to go, and how fast you want to get there. Simply take your dogs on an excursion and enjoy their company. There are no rules and no hurry, except the weather and your own time limits. You can explore new areas and even camp, if you wish.

You should have one dog trained as a lead dog. Once your lead dog is trained, you should train your other dogs in the basics of pulling. They should know the commands, "Hike!", "Whoa!", and "Tighten-up!" Unless you have experienced sled dogs, you should only add dogs to the team very slowly. Most new dogs have difficulty with the gang line and quickly become tangled. Should you have a tangle, stop the team immediately and untangle it. A tangled dog can injure himself or others and this may lead to a fight if the dogs become frightened. Likewise, never drag a dog. A dragged dog can be seriously injured or even killed.

Begin your training in the fall, when the weather turns cooler. Dogs overheat quickly in warm weather–a good rule is not to run a team when it is warmer than 50 degrees. In some areas, this may be prohibitive to mushing or the dogs must be specially conditioned for the weather. In Alaska, for example, dogs may overheat above 35 degrees. In some areas of the continental United States, mushers run their sled dogs in temperatures above 50 degrees. In any case, watch for signs of heat exhaustion and take frequent water breaks.

Start training by going only a half-mile every day for a week. Practice stopping and getting off the sled or cart. Be certain to properly tie-off the sled or cart with a snub line to prevent

Part 4

unexpected departures. Offer a quick treat to each of the dogs. As your dogs become used to your commands and control, they will become more reliable. Do not hook up more dogs than you can reasonably control. For most people, this is four dogs. As you gain experience, you can add dogs, provided that they are already harness-trained.

After the first week, you will increase to running one mile every day. As the days turn cooler and your dogs become more conditioned, you can take fewer breaks. Each week, you should double the mileage until you reach one mile per dog in the team. If you have four dogs, by the end of a month, you should be running four miles. At that point, you can train two to four times a week until racing season.

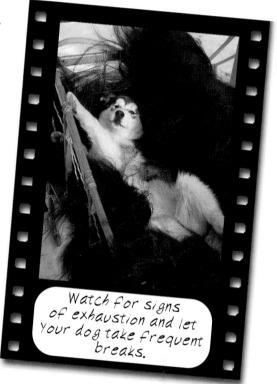

Watch for signs of exhaustion and let your dog take frequent breaks.

Part 4

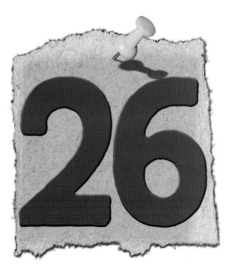

Traveling with Your Dog

If you become very involved in any of the activities or sports mentioned in this book, inevitably you'll decide to travel with you dog. Before you hop in the car or book that airline flight, you must make some important preparations. Traveling with your dog is often a major undertaking–dogs are not welcome everywhere. You must do your research in advance, including whether or not your lodging accepts pets, where you can eat with your canine companion, if your dog can accompany you to public places (like parks, beaches, tourist sites, etc.), and airline regulations regarding pets.

Health Certificates

Airlines require health certificates and advance notice if you and your canine friend are planning on

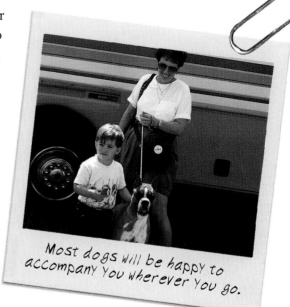

Most dogs will be happy to accompany you wherever you go.

taking to the friendly skies. You must obtain a health certificate within ten days of your travel date. If your return trip is more than ten days after the first health certificate is issued, you will need another health certificate. Only a veterinarian can issue health certificates.

Be certain that your dog's vaccination records are up to date and carry a copy of these records while traveling. If you are planning a trip in the country, ask your veterinarian about Lyme and giardia vaccinations for your dog. If fleas and ticks are a problem in the area you are entering, ask your veterinarian for recommendations for flea and tick control. Likewise, if you are planning a trip to a heartworm-prevalent area, ask for a heartworm test and preventative for your pet. Be aware that some dewormers and pesticides do not mix, so always consult your veterinarian before using them.

Airline Travel

Contact the airlines directly when you schedule your trip and tell them that you are taking your dog with you. The FAA has regulations regarding the shipment of animals; however, each individual airline has its own regulations and procedures. Airlines charge a fee for dogs on planes. Also, many have temperature restrictions that determine the times that animals can fly. Dogs that cannot fit in a carrier under the seat will have to ride in a crate in the baggage compartment. Most newer planes have pressurized and climate-controlled compartments, but this depends on the aircraft. Ask whether the baggage compartment is pressurized and climate controlled. This is important for your dog's safety as well as his comfort.

Even if the airline does not have temperature restrictions and the baggage compartment is climate controlled, you should be

Doggy Downers?

In case your dog becomes nervous or sick while traveling, ask your veterinarian if he can recommend tranquilizers. Be careful though! Some tranquilizers such as acepromazine can cause a dog with epilepsy to have seizures.

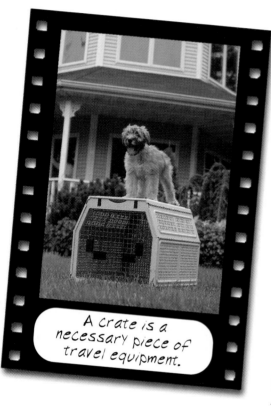

A crate is a necessary piece of travel equipment.

Part 4

mindful of the temperature. Sometimes dogs' crates are left on the ramp in blistering hot or freezing weather. Some baggage areas are not air-conditioned during the summer and may be too hot for your pet. If you must travel in the summer, do so at night or during the early morning hours when the temperature may not be so severe. In the winter, unless you have a Northern breed, be extremely careful of the temperatures outside and provide a blanket or other insulation. *Always book a nonstop flight* if one is available and avoid trips that require switching aircrafts.

Your dog will have to fly in a crate or carrier approved for airline travel. It must have dishes for water and food and be clearly marked that it carries a live animal. There are other regulations regarding crates, so contact the airline for their requirements.

Before you fly, photocopy your dog's health certificate and vaccination papers and slip them in a page protector taped to the top of your dog's crate. Keep the originals–you will need to show them at the airport.

Supply written information giving your dog's name, your address, phone number, destination, destination address and phone, veterinarian's name, medications needed, emergency numbers, the last time your dog was fed and watered, and when it is appropriate to feed or water your dog. Slip that into the page protector as well, face out so the baggage handlers can read it. A typical note might read: "Hi! My name is Sasha. I'm a purebred Alaskan Malamute. I am very friendly. I am flying with my owner John Jones to Denver, CO (DIA) on United Flight 1234 on Saturday, May 5, 2001 and returning home to

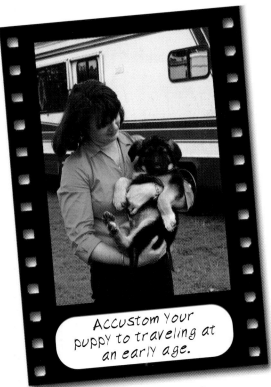

Accustom your puppy to traveling at an early age.

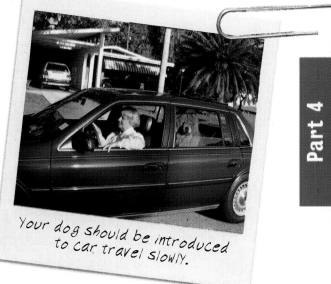

Your dog should be introduced to car travel slowly.

Minneapolis, MN on Sunday, May 13, 2001. My destination address is 123 Main Street, Parker, CO 80123; Phone number: (303) 555-1212. My veterinarian is Dr. John Smith at Lakeside Veterinary Clinic, St. Paul, MN. His number is (123) 456-7890. Contact Sarah Jones in case of emergency at (303) 555-1212. I do not need to be fed for 24 hours. I had water at the airport and do not need water until 6 pm MDT May 5, 2001. Copies of my health certificate and vaccinations are in this package."

Leaving on a Jet Plane

Listed below is some helpful travel tips from the Animal and Plant Health Inspection Service (APHIS), an agency of the US Department of Agriculture. The APHIS enforces regulations ensuring that animals traveling by air are treated humanely by airlines.

• If you are sending your pet through the cargo system, you will need to go to the airline cargo terminal, which is usually located in a separate part of the airport. Be sure to check with your airline for the acceptance cutoff time for your flight. By regulation, an animal may be present for transport no more than four hours before flight time (six hours by special arrangement).

• Use direct flights whenever possible to avoid accidental transfers or delays.

• Remember that some dogs are more likely to experience breathing problems during air travel, such as long-nosed dogs like Collies and pug-nosed breeds like Bulldogs.

• Attach instructions for feeding and watering an animal over a 24-hour period must be attached to the kennel. The 24-hour schedule will assist the airline in providing care for your animal in case he is diverted from his original destination.

• Carry a leash with you so that you can walk your pet before check-in and after arrival. Do not place the leash inside the kennel or attach it to the outside of the kennel—keep it with you.

• Outfit your pet with a sturdy collar and two identification tags. The tags should have both your permanent address and telephone number and an address and telephone number where you can be reached while traveling.

• Attach a label on the pet carrier with your permanent and travel addresses and telephone numbers.

• Make sure your pet's nails have been recently clipped to prevent snagging on the carrier door or other openings.

• Carry a current photograph of your pet. If your pet is accidentally lost, this will make the search easier.

• Don't be afraid to speak up. Let the crew know that your pet is traveling with you and that his safety is crucial.

If you need to file a complaint regarding the care of your pet during transport, contact the USDA-APHIS-Animal Care at (301) 734-4981.

Car Travel

Traveling with your best friend by car can be an enjoyable experience or a nightmare, depending on your preparation. First, be certain that your dog enjoys car rides. A dog that becomes carsick or hates riding in the car might be better off left at home with a pet sitter or in a boarding kennel. Likewise, a dog that is not housetrained or one that is poorly trained should not accompany you on a road trip.

Sometimes your destination precludes bringing a dog. Many vacation places have little or nothing to offer dogs and their owners. If you have any concerns about taking your canine companion to a particular vacation spot, find out what the area has to offer. If it has very little, consider another destination or board your dog. For example, many national parks do not allow dogs in the backcountry.

One rule that is often belabored but cannot be stressed enough is this: Never leave your dog in a car during the summertime–*even with the windows cracked.* Temperatures can soar inside the car within minutes and your dog can quickly suffer heat prostration and die. Your dog can also become overheated in crates, campers, and tents left in the sun.

Don't allow your dog to ride loose in the car. Crate your dog in your car to prevent him from distracting your driving and causing an accident. A crated dog is also a more comfortable dog–he will feel more secure in a crate.

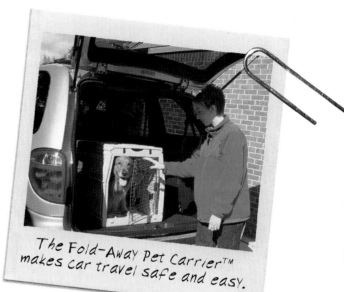

The Fold-Away Pet Carrier™ makes car travel safe and easy.

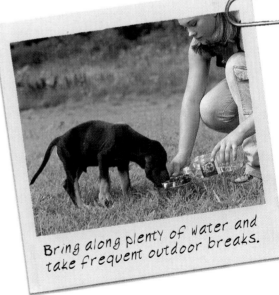

Bring along plenty of water and take frequent outdoor breaks.

Part 4

Never carry your dog in the back of a pickup truck. Every year, dogs are tossed from pickup beds with devastating results. If you have a pickup, put a top on it and crate your dog there. Open the side windows and check on your dog often to prevent overheating. However, do not open the back hatch window! Opening that window can pull exhaust in and can quickly poison your dog with carbon monoxide.

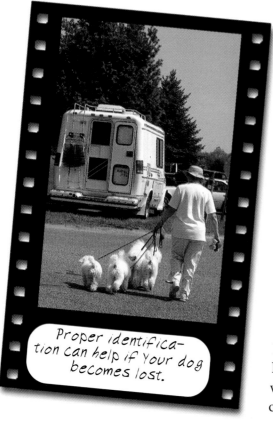

Proper identification can help if your dog becomes lost.

Equipment Checklist

The following is an equipment checklist for the well-traveled dog:

√ Travel crate

√ Dog food (include enough for two extra days)

√ Water bottle with enough water for the trip (some dog's stomachs become upset over changes in water)

√ Travel bowls for both food and water

√ Any medications your dog takes (including tranquilizers for the trip)

√ First aid kit

√ Travel toys

√ Blanket for dog to sleep on

√ Leash

√ Collar with identification

√ Recent photos—in case your dog becomes lost

√ Your veterinarian's emergency phone number and the emergency phone number of a veterinarian or animal hospital in the area you are traveling to.

√ Poop bags—for easy clean-up

Preventing the Unthinkable

Your vacation or trip with your best friend should be an enjoyable one. However, a lost dog can quickly turn your vacation into a nightmare. Keep your dog on a leash *at all times*, regardless of how well trained he is. Dogs often do not act the same on the road as they would at home, so be prepared. One moment off-leash could spell disaster.

However, even with the most vigilant owners, accidents do happen. Your dog might slip out of the motel when you open the door or might barge his way out of the car door before you can get the leash on. It is very important for your dog to have proper identification on him at all times.

Collar and Tags

The simplest form of identification is a collar and tags. Your dog's collar should be a flat collar (with a buckle or Fastex-type snap). Along with a rabies tag and a license, there should be an identification tag that gives your name, address, and phone number. These tags are inexpensive and available through mail order, veterinarians, tag engravers, and even pet stores. Many of the large pet supply stores now have tag-engraving machines that can produce a tag right there as you shop for dog food. These tags are cheap insurance in case your dog ever gets lost. If you are traveling for an extended period, you may wish to have a temporary tag with information on where you will be while traveling.

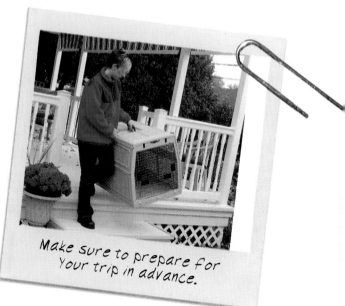

Make sure to prepare for your trip in advance.

As useful as collars and tags are, they do have their downsides. One is that the collar or tags can accidentally be pulled off while the dog is loose. If your dog is stolen, the thieves can remove the collar easily enough. Collars and tags are a quick way of identifying your dog, but they should not be the only method. You should always have a secondary form of permanent identification on your dog; that is, a tattoo or microchip.

Tattoos

Tattoos are a form of permanent identification. Unlike the collar and tags, which can be easily removed, the tattoo is a permanent mark, usually on the inside thigh. They are relatively inexpensive, especially if the tattoo is administered at a dog club sponsored event. Another good reason to tattoo your dog is that the law requires animal laboratories to check for tattoos on pets and prohibits them from using tattooed animals.

Tattoos are on file with a national registry such as National Dog Registry, Tattoo-A-Pet, or

Part 4

First Aid Kit

Dog first aid kits are a necessity, especially while you are traveling. Include the following in your dog's first aid kit:

√ Large and small nonstick bandage pads

√ Sterile gauze wrappings

√ Sterile sponges

√ Pressure bandages

√ Self-adhesive wrap

√ Disposable latex gloves

√ Triple antibiotic ointment or nitrofurizone (nitrofurizone is available through veterinary supply catalogues)

√ Bandage tape

√ Surgical glue (available through veterinary supply catalogues)

√ Cortisone cream

√ Muzzle

√ Rectal thermometer

√ Unflavored pediatric electrolyte

√ Syrup of ipecac™

√ Betadine solution

√ Bandage scissors

√ Petroleum jelly

√ Mineral oil

√ Kaolin product

√ Aspirin

√ Hydrogen peroxide

√ Tweezers

√ Your veterinarian's phone number, pager, and after-hours number

√ An emergency veterinary hospital's phone number where you are traveling

√ National poison control center phone number

Home Again. Tatoos are painless, but require that the dog must lie still while they are administered–something many dogs do not like. You must think up a unique number for the tattoo–many people use their social security numbers. This is fine, as long as you never intend to sell the dog! Owners who have tattooed dogs must keep the area free from hair so that the tattoo is readable. Occasionally, a dog may become allergic to the tattoo dye or the tattoo marks may fade or become unreadable. Dogs should not be tattooed in the ear–dog thieves can cut the ear off.

Microchips

The microchip is another way of permanently identifying your dog. Microchips are small pieces of circuitry in a container no larger than a grain of rice. They are relatively new. The chip's permanent number is read when a scanner is passed over it. The veterinarian or technician calls the registry that checks the number in a database and reads the corresponding owner's data. Microchipping your dog is a quick procedure–it takes about the same amount of time as a vaccination. The chip is injected between the shoulder blades and remains permanent unalterable identification.

The microchip may be relatively expensive compared to other options. There are several microchip manufacturers that require their own scanners and registries. Because microchips are invisible to the eye, a person who finds a dog may not know the dog is microchipped and may not have access to a scanner to determine if the dog was chipped. Not all shelters are equipped with microchip readers, and those that are may only be able to read one or two kinds of chips. Some microchip manufacturers such as Home Again are providing scanners at low or no cost to shelters. However, many veterinarians do have scanners and often aid in reuniting dogs and owners.

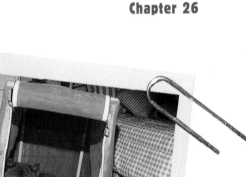

Most dogs can get comfortable wherever you stay.

If you decide to go with a microchip, be certain to choose a popular brand such as AVID or Home Again. Ask your veterinarian which microchip you should choose for your dog.

Where to Stay

Before you begin your trip, make reservations at a dog-friendly campground, hotel, or motel. If you arrive at your destination without a reservation, you may find there are no places to stay that accept pets. Many that do accept pets often have a size limitation or an additional fee.

Never try to sneak your dog into your lodging. Besides setting a bad precedent, you cannot hide a dog from hotel and motel staff. Aside from losing your money and being evicted, the facility may not be inclined to admit pets in the future.

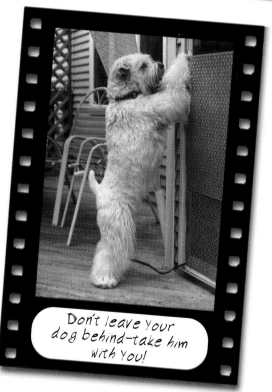

Don't leave your dog behind—take him with you!

Part 4

Proper Dog Etiquette

- Clean up after your dog. Always clean up after your dog defecates—no matter where you are! Even if you are in a pet exercise area, clean up after your dog! Set an example.
- Crate your dog. When you are unable to watch your dog, keep him crated. This prevents accidents and destructive behavior and will keep your dog safe.
- Clean up dog hair. Always pick up dog hair when you stay in a hotel or motel. Some pet owners bring a hair pickup roll to clean up after their pets.
- Don't leave your dog alone to howl or chew on furniture, or you won't be welcomed there again.
- Keep your dog on a leash. Never allow your dog to run loose. He may become lost. Well-trained dogs can sometimes forget their manners in strange places. Even if there is no leash law, keep your dog on a leash at all times.

Hotels and Motels

Contact the hotel or motel directly for reservations, because many do not allow pets. When you make reserv-ations, ask about the hotel's or motel's requirements. Many require that you do not leave your dog alone in the room and that you clean up after them. Keep your dog crated when you can to minimize dog hair and possible messes. Bring a blanket or sheet so that your dog's hair will not get into the bedding.

If your dog is quiet while crated in the room, you may be able to leave him for a short period of time while you eat dinner. However, many dogs, un-familiar with the strange surroundings, may bark and disturb the other guests. If there is a doubt, you may have to leave your dog in the car–provided it is not warm out. Remember that interior temperatures within a car can soar in the sun–even with the windows down. If the hotel has room service, you may wish to take advantage of it. This will allow you to eat with your dog, instead of locking him in a crate or in the car while you have dinner.

Don't bathe your dog in the tub or use the hotel's towels to dry off your dog. Don't leave your dog alone in the hotel room to chew and tear up furniture or soil the carpet. Remember that you and your dog are ambassadors for responsible dog ownership. If your dog is ill-mannered, it is unlikely the hotel will allow dogs again.

Campgrounds

Many campgrounds are still open to dogs; however, you should always contact the caretakers to find out what the rules are. Treat campgrounds as you would any motel or hotel. Don't leave your dog in the tent or camper to bark while you are gone, or you may not be welcome again. Don't allow your dog to run loose through the campground and disturb other campers who may not want a dog in their outdoor experience.

Be careful about leaving a dog alone in a tent in the summertime. Like cars, temperatures can soar within a tent and cause heat stroke.

Pet Sitters

If you can't take your pet with you when you travel, you can hire a pet care provider to come to your house once or twice a day to feed, walk, and play with your pet. The best part about this type of service is that your animal gets to stay at home where he feels most comfortable and can keep his daily routine.

When hiring a pet sitter, interview several candidates before making a decision. Remember that this person will have the responsibility for both your pet and home, so making the right selection is important. You should find out if the pet sitter is bonded, has commercial liability insurance, and will provide references. Ask for documented proof of these and check references.

Sitter Tips

To make sure everything runs smoothly while you're away, advanced planning is recommended. The following tips should help your pet sitter better care for your puppy:

• Make an extra copy of your house key for the sitter—and make sure it works. As a backup, give another copy of the key to a neighbor. Let your sitter know the name and phone number of this neighbor.

• Buy extra food and supplies just in case you stay away longer than anticipated.

• Leave a list of phone numbers, such as your veterinarian and the place where you are staying while away.

• All food, leashes, and medicines should be left in one area so they are easy to locate.

• If the sitter will be visiting in the evenings, provide a timer light so he or she won't have to walk into a dark house. It will probably make your pet more comfortable as well.

• If you will be returning earlier or later than expected, call to inform your sitter.

• Unplug any appliances that won't be used to prevent damage during electrical storms or injury to pets.

Part 4

Services offered and fees charged can vary widely depending on what state or town you live in. In a survey done by the National Association of Professional Pet Sitters, whose goal is to bring credibility to this fast-growing profession, the average charge is $10.00 per visit.

Once you've hired a sitter, let him or her know your puppy's daily eating, sleeping, and exercising schedule. Health problems should also be disclosed, as well as any medication your pet takes.

Boarding Kennels

Placing your pet in a boarding kennel is another option if you must travel for an extended period of time. Family, friends, co-workers, and your veterinarian are all good places to start your search for a well-run boarding kennel. Find out what they liked and disliked about the establishment, as well as how long they've used the facility or use the resources available to find licensed boarding kennels throughout the US.

Once you have some leads, make an unannounced visit to check out the facility. The first place you'll want to see is where the animals are kept. If you're not allowed to view this area, find another place. A reputable operator should never have a problem with showing the facility to a potential client. It could indicate a disorganized, unkempt place.

As you tour the kennel, you'll want to take note of a few things. The fencing used for cages or runs should be in good shape and smooth, with no sharp edges. There should be a solid barrier between cages that's high enough to prevent physical contact and cross urination. Also, if you have an escape artist dog, make sure the runs have covers and that the bottom of the fences is secure. The sleeping area of a run should be roomy enough for your pet to stand up comfortably, turn around in, and easily stretch out.

Overall, the facility should be clean, well lit, and odorless. Kennels should be disinfected daily with a cleaning solution, like diluted bleach, then rinsed thoroughly and allowed to dry before an animal is let back into the run to prevent chemical burns. The temperature should be set to a comfortable level. There should also be a good ventilation system, which allows fresh air to circulate into the kennel area.

While touring the facility, find out how often the dogs are checked during the day and if there is a play area for exercise. Some places will allow friends or family members to stop by and walk your dog while he is boarding. Also, check to see if your dog will have his own run or will be sharing it. A good kennel should honor the request for a dog to be boarded alone.

Ask what brand of food is fed. Some facilities only stock one type, while others have several popular varieties in order to match their clients' regular fare. If they don't have your dog's brand, find out if you can bring in a supply to be fed. Sticking with your dog's regular diet is important, because a sudden change can cause an upset stomach and/or diarrhea.

Inquiry about how they handle health situations and veterinary procedures. What is their policy if the kennel staff notices any health problems, such as vomiting, dehydration, bloody stool or urine? Will they take your pet to his regular veterinarian or use their own?

Check into which methods of payment they accept and their hours of operation. Some facilities might be closed on weekends and certain holidays, which means if you return home on those days, you won't be able to pick up your pet until the next day.

Usually boarders are required to be vaccinated for rabies, distemper, parvovirus, hepatitis, leptospirosis, parainfluenza, (the DHLPP vaccine) and bordetella or kennel cough. Ask if there are any other types of vaccinations required and what proof you'll need to show that your dog has the proper immunizations.

After your visit and before making a decision on what facility to use, take into consideration if the staff was friendly and if the business establishment was well run and organized. The more you know about the facility, the easier your mind will be about your puppy's welfare while you are away.

Part 4

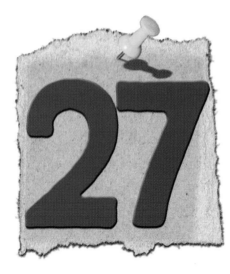

Conclusion

I've intended this book to be a guide for the novice on the variety of sports and activities available to the dog owner. Hopefully, you will come across one or two that will pique your interest enough to try it out. Dogs that do not do well in competitive obedience often have more fun in other sports and activities. If one does not appeal to you or your dog, try another. You'll eventually find something that you both will enjoy.

Although I have included basic training for each activity, I have not intended this book to be a substitute for training with a class. Training can greatly improve your success and allow you to enjoy your dog. Also, trainers and mentors are vitally important–they can show you the correct way of

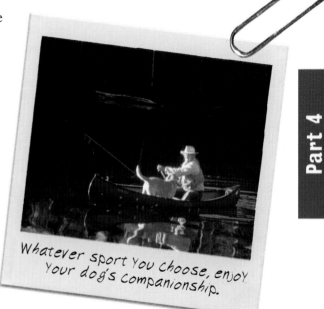

Whatever sport you choose, enjoy your dog's companionship.

training and point out possible pitfalls. Learning from others' mistakes, rather than make them over again, will make the learning process easier and less frustrating for both you and your dog.

The most important thing is to have fun with your dog and have a good time!

Part 4

Resources

General Information

American Kennel Club (AKC)

Headquarters:

260 Madison Avenue

New York, NY 10016

Operations Center:

5580 Centerview Drive

Raleigh, NC 27606-3390

Customer Services:

Phone: 919-233-9767

Fax: 919-816-3627

Web site: www.akc.org/

Email: info@akc.org

United Kennel Club, Inc. (UKC)

100 East Kilgore Road

Kalamazoo, MI 49002-5584

Phone: 616-343-9020

Fax: 616-343-7037

Web site: www.ukcdogs.com/

The Kennel Club

1 Clarges Street

Picadilly, London WIY 8AB, England

Web site: www.the-kennel-club.org.uk

The Canadian Kennel Club

89 Skyway Avenue

Suite 100

Etobicoke, Ontario, Canada M9W 6R4

Web site: www.ckc.ca

The Association of Pet Dog Trainers

17000 Commerce Parkway

Suite C

Mt. Laurel, NJ 08054

(800) PET-DOGS

information@apdt.com

Agility

Agility Association of Canada (AAC)

RR #2

Lucan, Ontario

N0N 2J0 Canada

519-657-7636

Web site: www.aac.ca/

Australian Shepherd Club of America (ASCA)

Lola Hill, Office Manager

PO Box 3790

Bryan, TX 77805-3790

Phone: 979-778-1082

Fax: 979-778-1898

Web site: www.asca.org

Email: lola@asca.org

United States Dog Agility Association, Inc. (USDAA)

PO Box 850955

Richardson, TX 75085-0955

Phone: 972-487-2200

Fax: 972-272-4404

Information Line: 888-AGILITY

Web site: www.usdaa.com/

Email: info@usdaa.com

Backpacking

Alaskan Malamute Club of America (AMCA)

Stephen Piper

3528 Pin Hook Road

Antioch, TN 37013-1510

Web site: www.alaskanmalamute.org

Email: cs@alaskanmalamute.org

Canine Backpackers Association LLC

PO Box 934

Conifer, CO 80433

Phone/fax: 866-728-7115

Web site: www.caninebackpackers.org

Email: skywarrior@juno.com

Canine Good Citizen®

American Kennel Club (AKC)

Headquarters:

260 Madison Avenue

New York, NY 10016

Operations Center:

5580 Centerview Drive

Raleigh, NC 27606-3390

Customer Services:

Phone: 919-233-9767

Fax: 919-816-3627

Web site: www.akc.org/

Email: info@akc.org

Carting

American Bouvier des Flandres Club, Inc.

David Raper

1718 Trinity Rd

Raleigh, NC 27607-4920

Web site: www.bouvier.org

American Rottweiler Club

Diane Garnett

4308 Whippeny Drive

Fort Collins, CO 80526

Web site: www.amrottclub.org/

Email: garnetts@worldnet.att.net

American Working Dog Federation (AWDF)

PO Box 523

Elizabeth, CO 80107

Web site: www.awdf.net/

Bernese Mountain Dog Club of America, Inc.

Mary Durham

P.O. Box 1158

Groton, MA 01450

Web site: www.bmd.org/bmdca.html

Email: mjd@bicnet.net

Newfoundland Club of America, Inc.

Robin Seaman, Corresponding Secretary

107 New Street

Rehoboth, MA 02769-2900

Web site: www.newfdogclub.org

Email: RSeaman985@aol.com

North American Working Bouvier Association (NAWBA)

Sheila Cronan, Secretary

3805 North 18th St.

Arlington, VA 22207

703-243-5842

Web site: www.nawba.org/

Email: scronan@erols.com

St. Bernard Club of America, Inc.

Marilyn Santell, Corresponding Secretary

735 G.P. Easterly NE

Cortland, OH 44410

330-637-9151

Web site: clubs.akc.org/saints/

Email: saintailkennels@aol.com

Conformation

American Kennel Club (AKC)

Headquarters:

260 Madison Avenue

New York, NY 10016

Operations Center:

5580 Centerview Drive

Raleigh, NC 27606-3390

Customer Services:

Phone: 919-233-9767

Fax: 919-816-3627

Web site: www.akc.org/

Email: info@akc.org

United Kennel Club, Inc. (UKC)

100 East Kilgore Road

Kalamazoo, MI 49002-5584

Phone: 616-343-9020

Fax: 616-343-7037

Web site: www.ukcdogs.com/

Flyball

North American Flyball Association, Inc.

1400 W. Devon Ave, #512

Chicago, IL 60660

309-688-9840

Web site: www.flyball.org/

Email: flyball@flyball.org

Flying Disc

Flying Disc Dog Open©

Bill Watters/Director

P.O. Box 4615

Cave Creek, AZ 85327

1-888-383-3357

480-595-0580 in Arizona

Web site: www.airmajorsdoghouse.com/fddo/

Email: director@fddo.org

National Canine Air Champions (NCAC)

The Washington D.C. Area FrisbeeTM Disc Dog Club

2830 Meadow Lane

Falls Church, VA 22042

703-532-0709

Web site: www.discdog.com

Email: ncac@discdog.com

Skyhoundz

4060 Peachtree Rd, Ste D #326

Atlanta, GA 30319

Phone: 404-256-4513

Fax: 404-256-9952

Web site: www.skyhoundz.com/

Email: info@skyhoundz.com

Freestyle

Canine Freestyle Federation

Monica Patty, Corresponding Secretary

21900 Foxden Lane

Leesburg, VA 20175

Web site: www.canine-freestyle.org/

Email: secretary@canine-freeestyle.org

World Canine Freestyle Organization Ltd.

PO Box 350122

Brooklyn, NY 11235-2525

Phone: 718-332-8336

Fax: 718-646-2686

Web site: www.worldcaninefreestyle.org

Email: wcfodogs@aol.com

Health

Canine Eye Registration Foundation

Department of Veterinary Clinical Science

School of Veterinary Medicine

Purdue University

West Lafayette, IN 47907

Phone: 317-494-8179

Fax: 317-494-9981

Web site: www.prodogs.com/chn/cerf/

Orthopedic Foundation for Animals

2300 E. Nifong Boulevard

Columbia, MO 65201-3856

Phone: 573-442-0418

Fax: 573-875-5073

Web site: www.offa.org

Email: ofa@offa.org

Herding

Australian Shepherd Club of America (ASCA)

Lola Hill, Office Manager

PO Box 3790

Bryan, TX 77805-3790

Phone: 979-778-1082

Fax: 979-778-1898

Web site: www.asca.org

Email: lola@asca.org

Hiking

Canine Backpackers Association LLC
PO Box 934
Conifer, CO 80433
Phone/fax: 866-728-7115
Web site: www.caninebackpackers.org
Email: skywarrior@juno.com

Lure Coursing

American Sighthound Field Association (ASFA)
Jack Helder, Corresponding Secretary
2975 Zimmer Rd.
Williamston, MI 48895
517-655-1173
Web site: www.asfa.org
Email: helder@paceandpartners.com

Mushing

Mush With PRIDE
Box 84915
Fairbanks, AK 99708-4915
Toll free: 1-800-50-PRIDE
907-457-6421
Web site: www.ptialaska.net/~pride1
Email: info@mushwithpride.org

Obedience

American Kennel Club (AKC)
Headquarters:
260 Madison Avenue
New York, NY 10016
Operations Center:
5580 Centerview Drive
Raleigh, NC 27606-3390
Customer Services:
Phone: 919-233-9767
Fax: 919-816-3627
Web site: www.akc.org/
Email: info@akc.org

United Kennel Club, Inc. (UKC)
100 East Kilgore Road
Kalamazoo, MI 49002-5584
Phone: 616-343-9020
Fax: 616-343-7037
Web site: www.ukcdogs.com/

Schutzhund

DVG America
Sandi Purdy, Secretary
2101 S. Westmoreland Rd.
Red Oak, TX 75154
972-617-2988
Web site: www.dvgamerica.com/
Email: SPurdy5718@aol.com

National Association of Protection Dogs (NAPD)

798 Hillborn Court

Suisun City, CA 94585

Phone: 707-422-5095

Fax: 707-422-5097

Web site: napdweb.org/

Email: NAPDSecty@aol.com

The United Schutzhund Clubs of America

3810 Paule Ave.

St. Louis, MO 63125-1718

Phone: 314-638-9686

Fax: 314-638-0609

Web site: www.germanshepherddog.com/

Search and Rescue

The American Rescue Dog Association

PO Box 151

Chester, NY 10918

Web site: www.ardainc.org

National Association for Search and Rescue

4500 Southgate Place, Suite 100

Chantilly, VA 20151-1714

Phone: 703-222-6277

Fax: 703-222-6283

Web site: www.nasar.org

Email: nasar@nasar.org

Sledding/Skijoring

Alaska Skijoring & Pulk Association

PO Box 82843

Fairbanks, AK 99708

Web site: www.sleddog.org/skijor

Email: patd@gci.net

Alaskan Malamute Club of America (AMCA)

Stephen Piper

3528 Pin Hook Road

Antioch, TN 37013-1510

Web site: www.alaskanmalamute.org

Email: cs@alaskanmalamute.org

International Federation of Sled Dog Sports (IFSS)

Sally Blair, IFSS Secretary General

16406 257th Avenue

Big Lake, MN 55309

Phone: 763-263-2818

Fax: 763-263-8471

Web site: www.sleddogsport.com/

Email: sblair@sherbtel.net

International Sled Dog Racing Association

HC 86 Box 3390

Merrifield, MN 56465

Phone: 218-765-4297

Fax: 218-765-3246

Web site: www.isdra.org

Email: dsteele@brainerd.net

Therapy Dogs

Therapy Dogs, Inc.
PO Box 2786
Cheyenne, WY 82003
307-638-3223

Therapy Dogs International
88 Bartley Road
Flanders, NJ 07836
Phone: 973-252-9800
Fax: 973-252-7171
Email: tdi@gti.net

Weightpulling

Alaskan Malamute Club of America (AMCA)
Stephen Piper
3528 Pin Hook Road
Antioch, TN 37013-1510
Web site: www.alaskanmalamute.org
Email: cs@alaskanmalamute.org

International Weight Pull Association (IWPA)
Dixie Smith, Membership
Phone: 406-257-4600
Fax: 406-257-0807
Web site: www.eskimo.com/~samoyed/iwpa
Email: ctn71350@centurytel.net

Travel Resources

Pet Sitters International
800-268-SITS

National Association of Professional Pet Sitters
1200 G Street, NW
Suite 760
Washington, DC 20005
800-296-PETS

The American Boarding Kennels Association
719-591-1113
http://www.abka.com

Periodicals

AKC Gazette
5580 Centerview Drive
Raleigh, NC 27606-3390
Customer Services:
Phone: 919-233-9767
Fax: 919-816-3627
Web site: www.akc.org/
Email: info@akc.org

Clean Run Productions, LLC

35 North Chicopee Street

Chicopee, MA 01020

1-800-311-6503

Outside the US: 413-532-1389

Fax: 413-532-1590

Web site: www.cleanrun.com/

Email: info@cleanrun.com

Dog Fancy Magazine

PO Box 53264

Boulder, CO 80322-3264

800-365-4421

Web site: www.dogfancy.com

Dog World Magazine

PO Box 56240

Boulder, CO 80323-6240

800-361-8056

Web site: www.dogworldmag.com/

Finish Line

Melanie McAvoy

1002 E Samuel Avenue

Peoria Heights, IL 61614

309-682-7617

Email: melmcavoy@worldnet.att.net

Front & Finish

PO Box 333

Galesburg, IL 61402-0333

Phone: 309-344-1333

Fax: 309-344-1165

Web site: www.frontandfinish.com

Mushing Magazine

Stellar Communications, Inc.

PO Box 149

Ester, AK 99725

Phone: 907-479-0454

Fax: 907-479-3137

Web site: www.mushing.com

Email: info@mushing.com

Team and Trail

PO Box 128

Center Harbor, NH 03226

Phone: 603-253-6265

Fax: 603-253-9513

Email: ttchbr@lr.net

Index

W

Photo Credits

Larry Allen: p. 95, bottom; p. 159.

Paulette Braun: p. 11, bottom; p. 14; p. 57; p. 58, bottom; p. 72; p. 76, top; p. 77, bottom; p. 78, bottom; p. 103; p. 163, bottom; p. 169, top.

Tara Darling: p. 106; p. 125; p. 128, bottom.

Isabelle Francais: p.9; p. 10; p. 11, top; p. 15; p. 17; p. 18; p. 19; p. 20; p. 21; p. 22; p. 23; p.24; p. 25; p. 26; p. 31; p. 32; p. 33; p. 34; p. 37; p. 39; p. 41; p. 42; p. 45; p. 46; p. 47; p. 51; p. 52; p. 53; p. 54; p. 58, top; p. 63; p. 65; p. 66; p. 69; p. 70; p. 73; p. 76, bottom; p. 78, top; p. 79; p. 80; p. 81; p. 82; p. 83; p. 84; p. 85; p. 86; p. 87; p. 88; p. 89, top; p. 93; p. 94; p. 95, top; p. 96; p. 97, bottom; p. 99; p. 101; p. 102; p. 105; p. 107; p. 108; p. 109; p. 113; p. 119; p. 120; p. 121; p. 123; p. 124; p. 127, bottom; p. 128, top; p. 129; p. 130; p. 131; p. 132; p. 133; p. 135; p. 136; p. 137; p. 138; p. 139; p. 142; p. 147; p. 149; p. 151; p. 153; p. 154; p. 155; p. 156; p. 157; p. 161; p. 162; p. 163, top; p. 165; p. 166; p. 169, bottom.

Honey Loring: p. 38

Alice Pantfoeder: p. 97, top;

Ron Reagan: p. 112;

Judith Strom: p. 64; p. 89, bottom; p. 90; p. 91; p. 117; p. 127, top; p. 141; p. 143; p. 144; p. 148; p. 152.

Karen Taylor: p. 40; p. 43; p. 44; p. 67; p. 75; p. 164; p. 167.

Cartoons by Michael Pifer